ELECTRICAL SAFETY IN
HEALTH CARE FACILITIES

CLINICAL ENGINEERING SERIES

Cesar A. Caceres, M.D., *Series Editor*

Clinical Systems Associates, Inc.

Washington, D. C.

Walmor C. De Mello. Electrical Phenomena in the Heart. 1972

Anthony Sances, Jr., and Sanford J. Larson. Electroanesthesia: Biomedical and Biophysical Studies. 1975

Herbert H. Roth, Erwin S. Teltscher, and Irwin M. Kane. Electrical Safety in Health Care Facilities. 1975

ELECTRICAL SAFETY IN HEALTH CARE FACILITIES

Herbert H. Roth

Instrumentation Consultant
Bioservice, Division of Teldicon, Inc.
Roslyn, New York

Erwin S. Teltscher

President
Bioservice, Division of Teldicon, Inc.
Roslyn, New York

Irwin M. Kane

Director of Engineering Services
Nyack Hospital, Nyack, New York
and
Adjunct Professor of Biomedical Instrumentation
Westchester Community College
Valhalla, New York

ACADEMIC PRESS   New York   San Francisco   London   1975
A Subsidiary of Harcourt Brace Jovanovich, Publishers

The authors have drawn upon numerous sources for the concepts and circuits described and have done their best to ensure the accuracy of all statements in this book. However, readers are advised to consult the technical literature provided by their equipment manufacturers in each case and to call upon competent technical personnel in applying the materials in this book to their particular equipment and electrical systems. In any case, neither the authors nor the publishers shall be liable or responsible in any manner whatsoever for any errors or omissions in this book.

ACADEMIC PRESS, INC.
111 Fifth Avenue, New York, New York 10003

United Kingdom Edition published by
ACADEMIC PRESS, INC. (LONDON) LTD.
24/28 Oval Road, London NW1

Library of Congress Cataloging in Publication Data

Roth, Herbert H.
    Electrical safety in health care facilities.

    (Clinical engineering series)
    Bibliography: p.
    Includes index.
    1.   Hospitals—Safety measures.   2.   Hospitals—Electric equipment.   3.   Medical electronics—Equipment and supplies—Safety measures.   I.   Teltscher, Erwin S., joint author.   II.   Kane, Irwin M., joint author.
III.   Title.   [DNLM: 1.   Accident prevention.   2.   Electric injuries—Prevention and control.   3.   Hospital equipment and supplies.   WX185 R845e]
RA969.9.R68   362.1'1'028   74-01217
ISBN 0-12-599050-2

CONTENTS

Chapter 4   The Characteristics of Installations

Chapter 5   Patient-Protection Systems

Chapter 6   Safety Testing

Chapter 7   Establishment of a Practical Safety, Preventive-Maintenance, and Repair Program

PREFACE

In the early nineteen seventies, numerous articles appeared in health care oriented publications dealing with electrical hazards in hospitals; these articles did not, however, provide a basis for gaining an understanding of the basic factors underlying any precautions taken to minimize such hazards.

This book, then, grew out of the need to explain in a systematic fashion why certain situations in hospitals are hazardous, how hazards can be minimized, and how to evaluate the many safety devices which have become available for improving hospital safety. Some of the material dealing with administrative matters has been necessarily based on the individual experiences of the authors. Technical material presented in this book has been kept simple, in order that it be readily understood by the audience it was intended to reach.

The authors gratefully acknowledge the cooperation in this effort of their wives, Trudy Roth, Florence Teltscher, and Minna Kane, without whose patience and assistance this work could not have been accomplished.

Herbert H. Roth
Erwin S. Teltscher
Irwin M. Kane

Chapter 1

INTRODUCTION

Only a decade or two ago, electrical hazards in hospitals were rare, and dangers from electricity were largely related to its potential for causing explosions in operating rooms. Today this picture has changed. It is true that the danger of explosion has been minimized by the use of nonexplosive anesthetics, but a new hazard has appeared on the scene. According to a recent article by Friedlander, the Food and Drug Administration has estimated that more than 1600 injuries and more than 100 deaths are caused by electrical equipment annually.

Why has this new problem arisen? The answer is twofold.

First, many new instruments have come into use. They have proven invaluable in providing better diagnosis and more effective treatment, but their use may cause side effects, such as electric shock, in certain categories of patients; these side effects are neither directly related to the use of the instruments nor readily detectable. Furthermore, the danger from electric shock that can occur when several such instruments are connected together has frequently not been assessed in advance.

Second, certain advanced techniques now being used, such as insertion of catheters into patients, are inherently dangerous when used in conjunction with instruments that have not been designed specifically to isolate the patient from virtually any possible electric shock, however minute it may be. For example, cardiac catheterization, if not carefully handled, can cause either mechanical or electrical injury to the heart, or even death. Cardiac arrest due to electric shock is, however, often indistinguishable from cardiac arrest due to other causes, especially in weakened patients, and can often be deduced only from circumstantial evidence.

What can be proved relatively easily, however, is whether hospitals provide a reasonably safe level of preventive maintenance and care to

1

ensure that there is very little chance of an electrical injury or accidental electrocution. The key words are "reasonably safe level of preventive maintenance and care." Why not absolute safety? Simply because absolute safety does not exist, but can only be approached—just as accidents cannot be absolutely eliminated, though their frequency can be reduced.

Everybody who works in a hospital, from the administrator and the physicians on down, is dedicated to the preservation of life, but the hospital also bears a heavy legal responsibility. Edgar Vanneman, Jr., a counsel to a medical-equipment manufacturer said recently: "The general legal rule is that the hospital has a responsibility to exercise ordinary care to furnish its patients, employees, and physicians a reasonably safe place. Thus, if an accident is caused because the electrical wiring in the hospital is faulty, because there is no common ground for the various outlets in the room, or because the wall plugs are faulty, this is a breach of [the hospital's] legal responsibility, and the jury is going to decide against [the hospital]."

The purpose of this book is, first, to provide a broad understanding of the principles underlying electrical safety in hospitals; second, to explain the factors that can cause electrical systems to become unsafe; and third, to outline appropriate procedures for maintaining safe electrical systems in hospitals and for organizing a safety and maintenance program.

Because of the varied background of people working in the health care field, such as administrators, doctors, nurses, engineers, and technicians, it was necessary to include some introductory material on electricity which can be read, for example, by administrators to help them to make necessary decisions, and by nurses and others to understand the rudiments of safe electrical practices. In the author's experience teaching courses on electrical safety to hospital engineering personnel it became clear that as a result of divergent educational backgrounds it was necessary to review basic principles of electricity even with members of that group.

Anybody approaching the subject for the first time and needing only a knowledge of its rudiments should at the minimum refer to the first part of Chapter 2, which provides a very basic introduction to electrical circuits and the terminology used elsewhere in the book. Those principles of electricity considered essential for properly understanding the operation of electrical and electronic equipment in hospitals are reviewed in the remaining part of the chapter, and are intended as a survey of such material. This will be particularly helpful to technicians and engineers who have not dealt extensively with the safe application of such equipment in hospitals, and to others who may wish to use it as a refresher course.

Chapter 3 discusses the electrical environment of the patient, the hazards to which a patient may become exposed, and the circumstances that may make him either more or less vulnerable to such hazards. This chapter will be particularly useful to doctors, administrators, and nurses, as well as engineers and technicians.

Chapter 4 discusses the characteristics of electrical installations, how to control voltage drops in ground wires, the effects of contacts, grounding systems for both instruments and installations, and the relation between a 3-phase supply and single-phase outlets. It will be of particular benefit to all those who must install electrical wiring in a hospital and to users of such electrical installations.

Chapter 5 deals with alternative systems and methods of patient protection.

Since hospitals, in general, vary widely in what precautions they have already adopted, improving safety becomes a matter of economics; those facilities that can be readily improved and upgraded will be retained, and only outdated equipment or installations that cannot be economically updated will be discarded. This applies not only to equipment but to hospital wiring systems which may not be up to standard, particularly in older hospitals. Various patient protection systems are discussed, and their applications, advantages, and possible disadvantages are reviewed. This chapter will be of particular help to all those who wish to improve the level of patient protection safety but have only a limited budget at their disposal and want to get the most for their money.

Chapter 6 deals with the important topic of how equipment is inspected and tested for safety. It will be of particular help to service department personnel charged with the responsibility of keeping equipment operable.

Chapter 7 reviews the relative advantages and disadvantages of contractor provided maintenance versus in-house safety and maintenance services. Examples of how considerable economies can be effected by setting up in-house safety and maintenance services are provided; ways and means of setting up a safety and maintenance department are discussed. This chapter will be of particular importance to hospital administrators facing a decision on whether to rely on contractor maintenance or whether to set up an in-house maintenance department.

Appendices were introduced to cover some rather specific and relatively technical topics for special applications. Since the authors have drawn upon numerous sources for the equipment, concepts, and circuits described, neither they nor the publisher can be liable in any way whatsoever for their application or for any errors or omissions herein, and the reader is advised to call upon competent technical personnel in applying these materials.

The book may be read in the sequence in which it is presented by the reader who first wants to acquaint himself with the broad outlines of the subject matter, or appropriate appendices may be read upon completion of pertinent sections of the book.

Bibliography

Friedlander, G. D., Electricity in Hospitals—Elimination of Lethal Hazards, *IEEE Spectrum* (Sept. 1971).

Vanneman, E., Jr., *Hospital* **43**, 118 (Sept. 16, 1969).

Chapter 2

BASIC ELECTRICITY AND HOSPITAL APPLICATIONS

This chapter introduces to the reader those basic principles of electricity required for an understanding of subsequent chapters. No equipment can be handled or operated safely without at least a rudimentary understanding of how it functions, how it can be interconnected, how it might affect a patient, and how to guard against dangerous malfunctions. It is the purpose of this chapter to acquaint the reader with only essential facts in the area, which are directly applicable to hospital safety.

The chapter is written in two parts. The first part provides a very basic introduction to electrical circuits and to the terminology used elsewhere in the book. The remaining part of the chapter is intended primarily as a survey of those principles of electricity considered essential for properly understanding the operation of electrical and electronic equipment in hospitals, and will serve as a review for some readers and as a guide to others. No prior knowledge other than high school mathematics is assumed.

Terminology and Fundamentals

Electric voltage or current is not directly observable by the human eye and can only be viewed with the aid of some instruments. The behavior of electric current is in many ways comparable to that of water flowing through a pipe. Imagine a long vertical pipe filled with water, the lower end of which is closed, for example, by a cap. Water will, of course, flow only if the cap is removed, and the flow of water will be proportional to the height of the pipe and to its cross section, i.e., the higher the water-filled pipe and the larger its cross section, the more water will flow out of it once the cap is removed.

The difference in height between the top and bottom portions of the water-filled pipe causes the water to be under pressure, and this is all really due to gravity. It is the pressure developed as a result of gravity that causes the water to flow out of the pipe, for if the pipe were suspended in a space ship, for example, where no gravity exists, no water would flow out. But pressure can also be exerted by a pump, for example, in a water-filled horizontal pipe, where the pump pressure would take the place of gravity.

To get a given amount of water to flow through the pipe, a given amount of pressure will have to be exerted. If the pipe is thin and long, more pressure will be needed than if the pipe is wide and short. Another way of looking at it is to say that a pipe which has a narrow diameter and is long will offer more resistance to water flow than a pipe which has a wide diameter and is short. There are direct analogies between water flowing through a pipe and electric current flowing through a wire. Water pressure corresponds to voltage: The stronger the water pressure, the more water will flow through a pipe; the greater the voltage, or potential, the more current will flow through a wire.

Resistance of a pipe to water flow and resistance of a wire to current flow are analogous quantities. The longer the wire and the smaller its diameter, the greater will be its resistance, and the more voltage will be needed to drive a given amount of current through the wire. Additionally, the amount of current flowing through the wire will also depend on the *type* of material used. While metals, for example, conduct electricity, not every material does, and even materials that are conductors offer varying degrees of resistance to current flow. The material most widely used is copper, since it conducts electricity very well. Nonconductors or insulators normally do not conduct electricity.

A wire connected to the positive and the negative terminals of a battery will conduct electricity, and may, for example, drive a motor or light a lamp. In the same way, a pump which keeps water moving through a pipe may drive a water wheel (Fig. 2-1). If the pipe is cut and both open ends are capped, water will cease to flow. Similarly, if the wire is cut, electric current will cease to flow, since cutting a wire and thus exposing it to contact with air is analogous to capping a pipe. In order to maintain a continuous flow of water through the pipe, continuous pressure must be applied by the pump to keep the water circulating. Likewise, a battery will have to supply a voltage continuously to keep the current circulating in the wire. In terms of water flowing through a pipe, the analogies with current

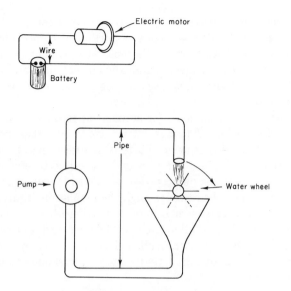

Fig. 2-1 Analogy of a pump driving a waterwheel with a battery driving an electric motor.

flow would be the following:

Water pressure is generated by a pressure source, e.g., a pump.

Voltage "pressure" is generated by a voltage source, e.g., a battery.

Water pressure keeps the water flowing in the pipe and causes work to be performed, i.e., the water wheel to turn.

Voltage keeps the current flowing and causes work to be performed, i.e., the electric motor to turn or the bulb to light.

Water flow must overcome the resistance of the pipe to its flow.

Current flow must overcome the resistance of the wire to its flow.

If the pipe is cut and the two resulting open ends of the cut pipe are capped, water ceases to flow.

If the wire is cut and the resulting two ends of the wire are capped by coming into contact with a nonconductor of electricity (such as air), current ceases to flow.

Turning a water wheel, lighting a bulb, driving an electric motor, and powering an electric heater are means to make the water—or electric current—perform work. Incidentally, when a bulb is lit by an electric current, only part of the work performed by the current is converted into light; the remaining part is converted into unwanted heat. Thus the bulb is not a very efficient converter of electric power into light. Similarly, many electric and electronic devices also convert part of the current they are consuming into unwanted heat, simply because they cannot be made to be 100% efficient in terms of converting all the current they are using to the particular end effect desired (such as showing a luminous trace of a heartbeat on an oscilloscope).

All analogies we have made so far correspond to direct current (or dc, its common abbreviation). The current we use in everyday life, however, is mostly alternating current or ac. There is no direct analogy with waterflow for alternating current, but it may be possible to conjure up one.

Imagine a pipe where the pump pressure exerted to cause the water flow varies periodically, i.e., the pressure might be high at one time, low after a certain time interval, and even negative—suction—later on, so that the water in the pipe would be alternately pushed forward and sucked back, its flow reversing cyclically. Although such a system has no practical application, the electrical analog of that system corresponds to the concept of alternating current.

Why is alternating current used in power-distribution systems instead of direct current? The use of alternating current has several advantages, one of the main ones being that a low voltage can easily be transformed into a high voltage via a transformer and thus be transmitted easily over long distances, and then be easily transformed again into a low voltage.

It will now be convenient to illustrate how an alternating voltage looks on an oscilloscope to examine its cyclical variation. The frequency at which an alternating power-line voltage varies cyclically has been established in the USA at 60 cycles per second or 60 hertz, abbreviated as Hz.* A typical 60-Hz voltage waveform is illustrated in Fig. 2-2. The time period denoted by T corresponds to one cycle of the waveform which oscillates at 60 Hz. T is equal in this case to $\frac{1}{60}$ sec or .0167 sec (commonly referred to as 16.7 msec). We are frequently interested in the amplitude of the waveform, i.e., the maximum excursion of the waveform from its center value which is termed the peak value of the waveform. A more frequently used term is the peak-to-peak value which is the maximum value of the waveform, as measured from the largest positive excursion to the largest negative excursion. The most frequently encountered term, however, is the root-

---

* Hereafter, standard abbreviations will be used for units of measure: seconds (sec), volts (V), amperes (amp), watts (W), etc. The prefixes m, μ, n, and p stand for milli (10^{-3}), micro- (10^{-6}), nano- (10^{-9}), and pico- (10^{-12}). Thus, 1 msec is 10^{-3} (or 1/1000) second, and so on. The only exception to this occurs when a prefix is added to the word "ampere." Then the abbreviation used will be A instead of amp, so that microampere will become μA.

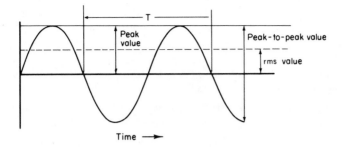

Fig. 2-2 Typical sinusoidally varying waveform for 60 Hz. $T = 1/60$ sec $= 16.7$ msec.

mean-square (rms) value which is equal to about 0.707 of the peak value of a sine wave (the alternating voltage waveform shown in Fig. 2-2). The rms value is sometimes called the *effective* value because it causes the same power dissipation in a load—such as in a light bulb—as would be caused by the same value of direct current or direct voltage. For example, a dc voltage of 110 V applied to a light bulb would cause it to glow with the same intensity as an rms ac voltage of 110 V; but the peak value of an rms voltage of 110 V is equal to about 155.6 V, and its peak-to-peak value is about 311.2 V.

Ohm's law states that in a circuit containing a resistance a voltage applied across that resistance will result in a current equal in value to the applied voltage divided by that resistance. This is shown in Fig. 2-3. The alternating voltage is denoted by V, the current by I, and the resistance by R (drawn by a zig-zag line as shown in the figure). Now Ohm's law applies to direct as well as to alternating currents. For example, if we apply a voltage of 110 V to a resistance of 110 ohms, the current flowing through that resistance will be 1 amp, resistance being measured in ohms and cur-

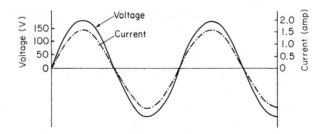

Fig 2-3 AC current produced when voltage is applied to a pure resistance of 100 ohms.

rent in amperes. If the resistance is 220 ohms, the current will be only $\frac{1}{2}$ amp. It is interesting to observe that the current will always be in phase with the voltage. This means that the peak excursion of the voltage will always coincide in time with a peak excursion of the current and that, when the voltage passes through a null point, the current will also pass through a null point.

In ac technology, we encounter occasions when the current is not in phase with the voltage, so that the peak excursion of the voltage does not correspond in time with the peak excursion of the current. This occurs when components other than resistances are used in a circuit. Examples of such components are capacitors and inductances denoted, respectively, by C and L, and symbolically drawn as shown in Fig. 2-4. The generic term "impedance" refers to the characteristics of an element in an ac circuit which may be either an inductance, a capacitance, a resistance, or a combination of these elements.

We can actually think of a current as flowing electric charges, for example, positive charges flowing from the positive battery terminal to the negative battery terminal. A capacitor is a device for holding such charges, similar to a tank holding water, and consists basically of two metallic plates separated by insulating material. If we connect such a capacitor across a battery, the capacitor would be charged with a certain amount of electric charges depending on its capacity to hold charges and would conduct current only as long as this charging process continues. Once it is fully charged, no current would flow. If, when the capacitor is charged, the battery is disconnected and the terminals of the capacitor are connected, the capacitor will discharge the stored electric charges in the form of a current which will last generally for only a very short time, i.e., until the capacitor is fully discharged.

In ac, however, where the applied voltage is continuously changing from zero to a positive value, back to zero, to a negative value, and back to zero again, a capacitor is constantly being charged and is in turn allowed to discharge, so that this can be visualized effectively as a current flowing through the capacitor. A capacitor connected in an ac circuit then can pass

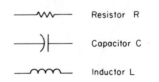

Fig. 2-4 Possible circuit elements of an impedance.

current, whereas in a dc circuit it cannot except for initial and terminal transient periods of very short, and generally insignificant, durations.

An inductance can be visualized as a device which, when a dc voltage is applied to it, permits the current to build up only gradually; in a resistance, however, the current reaches its assigned value immediately as soon as a voltage is connected across it. An inductance initially tends to resist a current flowing through it, although once a current is established in it, the current will generally continue to flow through it. If the current is interrupted, however, such as by cutting the connection to the voltage source (the battery), a spark will occur, depending on the magnitude of the applied voltage through which the current attempts to flow, even though the connection has been broken. Such a spark will, however, last for only a very short time. Except for the initial and terminal transient periods, an inductance connected in a dc circuit will behave just like a resistance, i.e., the resistance offered by the particular inductance connected in the circuit.

In ac circuits, an inductance can be visualized as an element with inertia which has the effect of delaying establishment of a current through it or, once a current is established, causing that current to decrease only gradually, even though the voltage which caused it to flow in the first place has already subsided to zero.

In ac circuits, then, the phase relationships between the voltage applied to a circuit element and the resultant current flowing in that element will depend on the nature of that element. In a resistor, the current will be in phase with the applied voltage; in an inductor, the current will lag behind the applied voltage; and in a capacitor, the current will lead the applied voltage. This is shown graphically in Fig. 2-5.

The value of an inductance is measured in units called henrys and the value of a capacitor in units called farads. Since the farad is, however, a

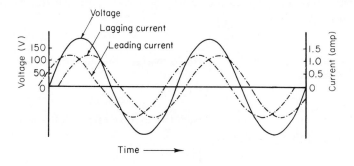

Fig. 2-5 AC current produced when voltage is applied to an impedance.

unit of a very large value, it is more common to use a unit one millionth of a farad, the microfarad.

A capacitor will be formed by any conducting objects such as, for example, wires in close proximity, although the value of such a capacitor will naturally be much smaller than the value of a capacitor specifically designed to hold a certain amount of electric charges. Nevertheless, the fact that any conducting objects in close proximity can form a capacitor is of importance in dealing with patients who for one reason or another are more vulnerable to small currents than a normal healthy person; for, if one side of such a capacitor is connected to an electric voltage source and the other side is connected accidentally to the patient, a current can pass through the patient if and only if a return connection from the patient to the voltage source also exists. Such a return connection, frequently caused by a ground connection, can exist, and this type of hazard is discussed in greater detail in Chapter 3. Unwanted currents through capacitors, formed spuriously and in the manner indicated, or through other elements, are generally called leakage currents, and the formation of unwanted leakage currents must be avoided to ensure safe conditions for electrically vulnerable patients.

The reader who wishes to continue his or her education in electricity more comprehensively through an easily understandable text before tackling the more advanced subject matter in this book can do so by consulting the sections dealing with electricity in *Physical Science in the Modern World* by J. B. Marion, or some other equivalent easily understandable reference book. The remaining sections in this chapter are recommended for readers who either have had some background in this subject already or are otherwise capable of handling a minimum amount of mathematics.

Ohm's Law, Impedance, and Vectorial Addition in AC Technology

Ohm's Law, briefly stated in the previous section, can be more concisely written as

$$V/I = R$$

or, if we introduce a term *admittance*, the inverse of resistance (i.e., equal to $1/R$), and denoted by G,

$$VG = I$$

Another important concept is power denoted by P. Most of us are familiar with the concept of horsepower (e.g., the horsepower developed by the motor of a car). Just as mechanical power can be developed, so can electrical power. The amount of power used or dissipated in an electrical resistive circuit is given by

$$P = VI$$

and is measured in watts; i.e., power is proportional to the product of voltage and current. But we already know that

$$V/R = I \quad \text{or} \quad V = IR$$

Substituting for V in the power equation, we obtain

$$P = I^2R$$

which means that the power dissipated in a resistance is proportional to the square of the current flow multiplied by that resistance. We could also have substituted for I in the power equation, in which case

$$P = V^2/R$$

All three expressions are equally valid, and power can be calculated from any of the expressions; which expression one chooses is simply a matter of convenience depending upon which quantities are known or are easiest to measure.

All of the foregoing quantities are applicable to both dc and ac; the relationship between current, voltage, admittance, resistance, and power is summarized in Table 2-1.

As has already been stated in the previous section, in ac technology we encounter occasions when the current is not in phase with the voltage, so that the peak excursion of the voltage does not correspond in time with the peak excursion of the current, as can be seen from Fig. 2-5. Whenever a

Table 2-1
Summary of Relationships between Current, Voltage, Admittance, Resistance, and Power[a]

I	V	G	R	P
VG	RI	I/V	V/I	I^2R
V/R	I/G	I^2/P	P/I^2	I^2/G
$(P/R)^{1/2}$	$(P \cdot R)^{1/2}$	$1/R$	$1/G$	V^2/R
$(P \cdot G)^{1/2}$	$(P/G)^{1/2}$	P/V^2	V^2/P	V^2G

[a] Expressions in vertical columns are equivalent.

current produced as a result of an applied voltage lags that voltage, we already know that an inductance must be present in the circuit, and conversely when the current leads that voltage, a capacitance will be present in the circuit. While a resistive element offers a resistance to the flow of current, an inductance or capacitance offers a reactance to the flow of current (the reactance, as we shall see later, being a function not only of the particular value of the inductance or capacitance of the element, but also of the frequency of the ac employed). Furthermore, a pure reactance does not consume any power; it merely recirculates the power from the source to that element. The element returns the power again to the source in each cycle of the ac wave, just as an ideal pendulum, which does not encounter any air or other resistance will theoretically oscillate forever.

Where a combination of a resistance and a reactance is used, the more general term *impedance* is employed, as has already been stated. Calculations are carried out more simply in terms of impedance rather than resistance, capacitance, or inductance. Since the impedance of a circuit is generally a function of the frequency of the applied voltage, the frequency must be brought into these calculations. The alternating voltage waveform of Fig. 2-1 can be expressed mathematically as

$$V = V_p \sin 2\pi f t$$

where V is the instantaneous voltage at any time t, V_p is the peak value of the voltage and is considered constant, and $2\pi f t$ is an angle, where π is the ratio of the circumference of the circle to its diameter and is approximately equal to 3.14, t is the instantaneous time in seconds, and f is the frequency in hertz, usually equal to 60 in calculations involving power lines. Sin $2\pi f t$ is then the sine of the angle $2\pi f t$. Since the sine of an angle can vary from $+1$ to -1, sin $2\pi f t$ will also vary from $+1$ to -1. Furthermore, instead of $2\pi f$ it is more convenient to use the symbol ω, so that the above expression can be simplified to read

$$V = V_p \sin \omega t$$

Since $f = 60$ Hz, $2\pi 60 \approx 377$, and the preceding expression reduces numerically, for a power supply varying at a frequency of 60 Hz, to

$$V = V_p \sin 377t$$

Referring again to Fig. 2-5, this means that if V_p, the peak value of the voltage is, for example, 100 V, then the value of V will increase from 0 to 100 V in one-fourth cycle or in approximately 4.2 msec at a frequency of 60 Hz, will decrease to zero in the next quarter-cycle, will turn to -100 V in the succeeding quarter-cycle, and will revert to zero volts at the end of the last quarter-cycle. In numerical terms the instantaneous voltage is written as

$$V_i = 100 \sin 377t$$

V_i denoting instantaneous voltage, and this expression will tell us at any given time what the instantaneous voltage will be.

What is the current in a 50-ohm resistor? Here it is legitimate to obtain the current by dividing the voltage by the value of the resistor; therefore, the instantaneous current I will be

$$I_i = V_i/R = (100 \sin 377t)/50 = 2 \sin 377t \text{ amp}$$

More generally, the instantaneous current in a resistor due to an alternating voltage will be given by

$$I_i = (V_p \sin \omega t)/R$$

and the current will at all times be in phase with the voltage applied across the resistor, as shown in Fig. 2-6.

Suppose now that this same voltage is applied across a capacitor; what current will flow through the capacitor? The extension of Ohm's law applicable to an impedance states that the current is equal to the applied voltage divided by the impedance.

It will now be stated without proof that the magnitude of the reactance offered by a capacitor is given by

$$Z = 1/\omega C$$

and furthermore that when an alternating voltage is applied across a capacitor, the current leads the voltage by 90°. The reader interested in understanding why this is so will find it explained in Appendix B.

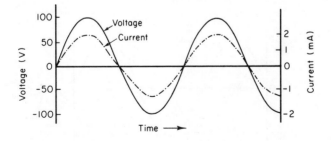

Fig. 2-6   Relationship between an applied ac voltage having a peak value of 100 V and current in a resistor of 50 ohms. The current is in phase with the applied voltage. The peak value of the current will be seen to be 2 amp, and its rms value $0.707 \times 2 = 1.41$ amp.

Taking a specific value of a capacitor, say 1 μF, the value of the reactance offered by the capacitor will be seen to be

$$Z = 1/(377 \times 1 \times 10^{-6}) = 2652 \text{ ohms}$$

The peak current I flowing through the capacitor as a result of applying a peak voltage of 100 V will then be

$$I_p = V/Z = 100/2652 = 0.0377 \text{ amp} = 37.7 \text{ mA}$$

This current, in relation to the applied voltage, is shown in Fig. 2-7. We notice immediately that the current leads the voltage by 90°. How do we know that the voltage is not lagging the current by 270°? Well, if we looked at Fig. 2-7 only, we could not tell the difference, but in fact for the simple case described above it will be stated without proof that the current flowing through a capacitor cannot lead the impressed voltage by more than 90°, and so we know that the current does in fact lead the impressed voltage.

Similarly, when current is flowing through an ideal inductor, i.e., an inductor which is assumed to have zero resistance, the magnitude of the impedance offered by the inductor is given by

$$Z = \omega L$$

When an alternating voltage is applied across an inductor, the voltage leads the current by 90° as shown in Fig. 2-8. This is explained in further detail in Appendix B.

Taking again a specific value of an inductance, say 1 henry, the value of the impedance will be seen to be

$$Z = 377 \times 1 = 377 \text{ ohms}$$

and the peak current flowing through that impedance with an applied ac

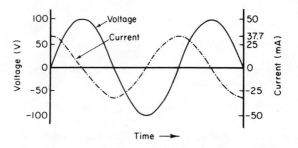

Fig. 2-7 Relationship between applied ac voltage and current in capacitor. The current leads the voltage by 90°.

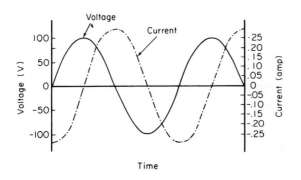

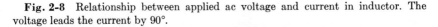

Fig. 2-8 Relationship between applied ac voltage and current in inductor. The voltage leads the current by 90°.

peak voltage of 100 V will be

$$I_p = 100/377 = 0.265 \text{ amp}$$

The rms value of the current will of course be in all cases 0.707 of its peak value.

A summary chart of the relationships just discussed is given in Table 2-2.

Voltages and currents can also be represented as vectors. Consider, for example, the two vectors shown in Fig. 2-9,* one vector representing a voltage, the other representing a current. If both vectors are now envisaged as rotating counterclockwise, their projection on the X-axis will be seen to vary sinusoidally from a positive maximum to a negative maximum. If the magnitude of the voltage vector is set equal to 100 V and that of the

Table 2-2
Current Flowing through Circuit Elements

Parameter	Resistor	Capacitor	Inductor
Z	R	$1/\omega C$	ωL
I	V/R	$V\omega C$	$V/\omega L$
Phase of current with respect to voltage	Same	Leading by 90°	Lagging by 90°

* The literature refers to alternating voltages and currents both as vectors and phasors. The term *phasor* is the more recent denotation. Strictly speaking, a vector represents a magnitude and a direction, whereas a phasor represents a magnitude and a time relationship to another phasor.

current vector to 37.7 mA, the sinusoidal variation of the voltage and current will be as shown in Fig. 2-7.

We are only very infrequently concerned with the exact value of a voltage or current at a given moment in time; what is of interest, however, is their relative phase and their peak and rms values. These parameters are conveyed just as well by the simpler vector diagram of Fig. 2-9, so that there is no need to always indicate the complete sinusoidal waveforms depicted in Figs. 2-5–2-7. An overall comparative view of a reference voltage and the currents produced by that voltage in a resistor, a capacitor, and an inductor appears in Fig. 2-10. These relationships are further discussed in Appendix B.

The voltages and currents we have discussed so far have been shown to be either in phase, or leading or lagging each other by 90°, because we have discussed only pure resistances, pure capacitances, and pure inductances. We do, however, encounter circuit constants that are mixtures of inductance and resistance, capacitance and resistance, or any other combination. In such cases we can obtain circuits in which the voltage lags the current by less than 90°, or leads it by less than 90°. This happens, for example, when a resistor is in series or in parallel with an inductor or a capacitor. Let us illustrate series and parallel connections with resistors.

Figure 2-11 shows two resistors in series. A common current I flows through both resistors; by Ohm's law, the voltage across resistor R_1 will be

$$R_1 I = V_1$$

and the voltage across resistor R_2 will be

$$R_2 I = V_2$$

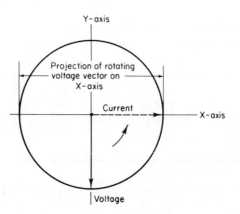

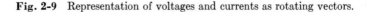

Fig. 2-9   Representation of voltages and currents as rotating vectors.

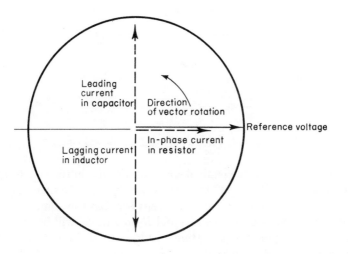

Fig. 2-10 Diagram comparing phase angles between applied voltage and resulting current in resistor, capacitor, and inductor.

The total voltage V_T across resistors R_1 and R_2 in series will be given by

$$V_T = V_1 + V_2$$

Figure 2-12 shows two resistors in parallel, with a common voltage V across them. A current I_1 flows through resistor R_1, and a current I_2 flows through resistor R_2; the current flowing into one junction and out of the other junction will be given by I_T, the total current, and will in fact be equal to $I_1 + I_2$.

The series resistors in Fig. 2-11 could be replaced by a single equivalent resistor R_{eq}, where $R_{eq} = R_1 + R_2$, which would yield the same current flowing in the resistor R_{eq} as flows in resistor R_1 and resistor R_2, and the same voltage V_T across R_{eq} as is obtained across the combination of resistors R_1 and R_2.

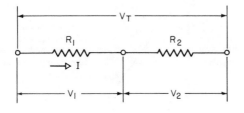

Fig. 2-11 Two resistors in series; $V_T = V_1 + V_2$.

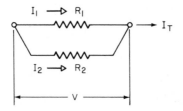

Fig. 2-12   Two resistors in parallel; $I_T = I_1 + I_2$.

How do we calculate the equivalent resistance R_{eq} in the case of the two parallel resistors of Fig. 2-12? Here the concept of admittance, the inverse of resistance, becomes useful. We can easily see that the admittance of the combined network of resistances R_1 and R_2 in parallel will be equal to the admittance of R_1 plus the admittance of R_2. But the admittance of R_1 is G_1, where $G_1 = 1/R_1$, and that of R_2 is G_2, where $G_2 = 1/R_2$. Hence, G_T the total admittance is equal to $G_1 + G_2$, and $R_{eq} = 1/G_T$. More specifically,

$$G_T = 1/R_1 + 1/R_2 = (R_1 + R_2)/R_1R_2$$

and

$$R_{eq} = 1/G_T = R_1R_2/(R_1 + R_2)$$

Substantially the same principle is used in working out the total impedance offered by a series or parallel combination of resistance and inductance or resistance and capacitance, the only difference being that we add the currents or voltages, not algebraically, but vectorially. To illustrate the concept of vectorial addition, consider a boat trying to cross a river at a speed of 4 knots when the river itself is flowing at a speed of 3 knots, as shown in Fig. 2-13. If the boat is aimed exactly toward the opposite shore of the river, it will in fact drift downstream while crossing, because of the downstream velocity of the current. Since the intended velocity of the boat

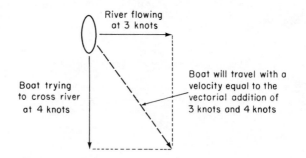

Fig. 2-13   The concept of vectorial addition.

and the velocity of the stream itself are at an angle of 90°, the two velocities must be added vectorially to arrive at the velocity and direction at which the boat will finally be traveling. This is shown graphically in Fig. 2-13. The final velocity of the boat will be given by $v = (4^2 + 3^2)^{1/2} = 5$ knots, and the angle at which the boat will deviate from its intended direction will be given by $\tan^{-1} \frac{3}{4}$, i.e., an angle whose tangent is $\frac{3}{4}$, or 0.75, which corresponds to an angle of 36°48'.

As we shall see later on, the calculation of a voltage across a resistor in series with an inductor is performed in a very similar manner. But before we actually perform such a calculation, it will be useful to show how such calculations can be systematized by the use of the operator j. The complexity of calculating, say, a voltage across the series combination of a resistor and inductor does not differ very much, whether we use the straightforward vectorial addition, as illustrated in the case of the boat crossing the river, with the river itself flowing downstream at a finite velocity, or whether we use the j operator; but for more complex configurations, the use of the j operator has a definite advantage and permits systematic calculations of any combination of impedances, voltages, or currents encountered.

The operator j is actually an imaginary number, and is equal to $\sqrt{(-1)}$; since there is no real number that, when squared, is equal to -1, we use the following identity: $j = \sqrt{(-1)}$, where j is an imaginary number. This imaginary number j has some definite properties, though; for example $j^2 = -1$. Also, we can convert any number containing several j's, or imaginary numbers, to a *complex number* containing a real part and an imaginary part only. As an example, consider the fraction

$$Z = (R_1 + jX)/(R_2 - jX)$$

This number can be easily converted to a number in the form

$$Z = A + jB \qquad \text{or} \qquad Z = A - jB$$

which two expressions can be combined to yield

$$Z = A \pm jB$$

This is much simpler than the fraction previously shown. The conversion is done in the following steps:

1. Multiply both numerator and denominator with the complex conjugate of the denominator. (The complex conjugate is a number identical with the number having a real and an imaginary part, except that the sign of the imaginary part is reversed.)
2. Multiply individual terms.

Table 2-3
Steps Performed in Calculating Real and Imaginary Parts of a Fraction Containing Complex Numbers

Step	Expression	Action
	$$\dfrac{R_1 + jX}{R_2 - jX} =$$	Write down fraction. Note that if denominator has the form $R_3 + jX$ complex conjugate is $R_3 - jX$.
(1)	$$\dfrac{(R_1 + jX)(R_2 + jX)}{(R_2 - jX)(R_2 + jX)} =$$	Multiply both numerator and denominator by complex conjugate of denominator, i.e., $(R_2 + jX)$ for the example shown.
(2)	$$\dfrac{R_1R_2 + jR_1X + jR_2X + j^2X^2}{R^2_2 - jXR_2 + jXR_2 - j^2X^2} =$$	Multiply individual terms.
	$$\dfrac{(R_1R_2 - X^2) + jX(R_1 + R_2)}{R^2_2 + X^2} =$$	Group real and imaginary terms. (Note that any j^2 terms are real terms, since $j^2 = -1$.)
(4)	$$\dfrac{R_1R_2 - X^2}{R^2_2 + X^2} + j\dfrac{X(R_1 + R_2)}{R^2_2 + X^2} =$$	Break down into real and imaginary terms.
(5)	$0.04 + j0.78 =$	Substitute given values, in this case using $R_1 = 5$, $R_2 = 8$, and $X = 6$ ohms.

3. Group together real and imaginary terms. Note that any terms prefixed by j^2 become real, since $j^2 = -1$.

4. Break down into real and imaginary terms.

5. Substitute the given values for the resistances and reactances involved. (Note that a reactance is an impedance that is purely imaginary—i.e., having no real component.)

An example of how these steps are performed is shown in Table 2-3. Note that the final result is a complex number having two terms—a real term and an imaginary term.

Consider now a series combination of a resistance R and an inductance L, with alternating current of magnitude I flowing through the combination; what will be the value of the voltage across terminals A and B of this combination, and what will be the vectorial relation of that voltage to the current I?

The voltage across the resistor will be RI, and that across the inductor will be $j\omega LI$, so that the combined voltage across the resistor and the inductor will be the vectorial summation of these two voltages, given by

$$V_{AB} = RI + j\omega LI$$

This looks simple enough, but does not tell us yet how many volts would appear across these terminals if we measured the terminal voltage with a voltmeter. The *absolute magnitude* of that voltage is given by the vectorial addition of these terms; it is equal to the square root of the square of the voltage across the resistor plus the square of the voltage across the inductor. The absolute magnitude of a voltage V is denoted by $/V/$; hence

$$/V_{AB}/ = [(RI)^2 + (j\omega LI)^2]^{1/2}$$

For example, if $I = 1$ amp, $R = 30$ ohms, and $L = 0.106$ henry, then $j\omega L = /40/$ ohms, so that

$$/V_{AB}/ = (30^2 + 40^2)^{1/2} = 50 \text{ V}$$

The phase angle by which the voltage will lead the current is now less than 90° and given by the angle whose tangent is $j\omega L/R = \tan^{-1}(40/30)$ or 53°12′. The vectorial addition of these voltages is also illustrated in Fig. 2-14.

Now consider the calculation of the impedance offered by the combination of a resistor and capacitor in parallel. As in the case of two resistors in parallel, this is best done by adding the admittances of the two branches. The impedance offered by the resistor is simply its resistance R; the impedance offered by the capacitor is equal to $1/j\omega C$, or $-j/\omega C$. Hence, the

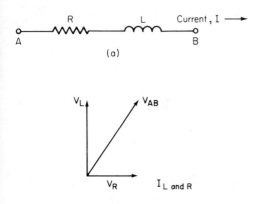

$$/V_{AB}/ = [(RI)^2 + (j\omega LI)^2]^{1/2}$$

Fig. 2-14   (a) Determination of the voltage across a series combination of a resistor and a capacitor by both calculation and vectorial addition. (b) Impedances are vectorially added in a series circuit. V_{AB} is the voltage across terminals A–B, $I_{L\&R}$ the identical current in both L and R.

admittance of the resistive branch will be $1/R$, and that of the capacitative branch will be $j\omega C$. Adding these two terms, the combined admittance of the circuit as seen across terminals E and F will be given by $G_{EF} = 1/R + j\omega C$. The impedance Z_{EF} will be the inverse of the admittance, or

$$1/G_{EF} = 1/(1/R + j\omega C) = Z_{EF}$$

Multiplying both numerator and denominator again by the complex conjugate of the denominator—i.e., by $(1/R - j\omega C)$—we obtain

$$Z_{EF} = (1/R - j\omega C)/[(1/R)^2 + \omega^2 C^2]$$

Again we can see that the impedance contains a real term and an imaginary term. For example, if $R = 50$ ohms and $C = 26.5$ μF, then $-j\omega C = j0.01$ mho (the unit of conductance) so that

$$Z_{EF} = (0.02 - j0.01)/[(0.02)^2 + (0.01)^2] = 40 - j20 \text{ ohms}$$

Again the absolute value of the impedance

$$/Z_{EF}/ = (40^2 + 20^2)^{1/2} = 44.7 \text{ ohms}$$

and the phase angle of the impedance with respect to a pure resistance is $\tan^{-1}(20/40) = 26°34'$. Since the imaginary part is negative, the phase angle of the impedance is lagging with respect to the phase angle of a pure resistance, as illustrated in Fig. 2-15.

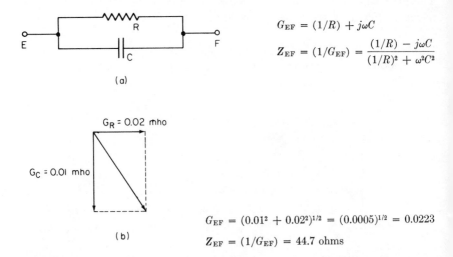

$$G_{EF} = (1/R) + j\omega C$$

$$Z_{EF} = (1/G_{EF}) = \frac{(1/R) - j\omega C}{(1/R)^2 + \omega^2 C^2}$$

(a)

$$G_{EF} = (0.01^2 + 0.02^2)^{1/2} = (0.0005)^{1/2} = 0.0223$$

$$Z_{EF} = (1/G_{EF}) = 44.7 \text{ ohms}$$

(b)

Fig. 2-15 (a) Determination of the impedance offered by a combination of a resistor and a capacitor by both calculation and vectorial addition. (b) Admittances are vectorially added in a parallel circuit; impedance = 1/resultant admittance.

We might legitimately ask what is the meaning of an impedance that has a leading or lagging phase angle. Since $V = IZ$, the voltage will lead or lag the current, depending on whether the phase angle of the impedance is leading or lagging.

It will be recalled that in dc technology, power is given by the product of current times voltage: $P = IV$. This concept must now be qualified in ac technology. $P = IV$ holds only when the phase angle between the current and the voltage is zero—i.e., when current flows in a pure resistance. When there is a phase angle θ between the applied voltage and the resultant current, the power P is given by

$$P = VI \cos \theta \text{ watts}$$

An interesting result of this equation is the fact that when a circuit element is purely inductive or purely capacitive, no power is dissipated in that circuit element over a long period; energy flows into the element in one part of the cycle, to be returned during the next part of the cycle.

Resonance

The use of a capacitance and an inductance in a circuit, either in series or in parallel, produces a condition termed resonance. Resonance occurs at a frequency where the positive reactance due to the inductance of a coil equals the negative reactance due to the capacitance of a capacitor, and is similar to the familiar resonance condition encountered when a tuning fork is struck and consequently emits sound at a particular pitch of frequency. By setting the inductive reactance equal to the capacitative reactance and solving for the frequency of resonance f_r, the following equation is obtained:

$$f_r = 1/2\pi (LC)^{1/2}$$

In practice, however, these ideal conditions can never be realized, since it is not possible to construct an inductor without resistance, and even the best capacitors have some finite leakage resistance. Nevertheless, the leakage resistance in a capacitor can usually be neglected in comparison to the resistance offered by an inductance, and therefore an approximation neglecting the leakage resistance of a capacitor will be valid in most cases. The ratio of inductive reactance ωL to resistance R in the inductor of a resonant circuit will determine the "quality" Q of the circuit. The higher this ratio $\omega L/R = Q$, the sharper the resonance of the circuit will be.

In a series resonant circuit, the impedance of the circuit will be lowest at resonance, equaling the resistance R of the coil at resonance. In a parallel

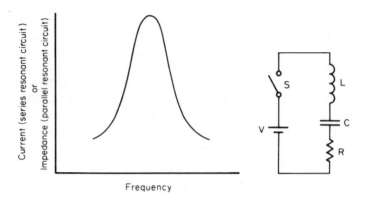

Fig. 2-16   Fig. 2-17

Fig. 2-16 Current variation of a series resonant circuit, or impedance variation of a parallel resonant circuit, as a function of frequency.

Fig. 2-17 Application of dc to series resonant circuit.

resonant circuit, the impedance of the circuit will be maximum at resonance and equal to L/RC.

The variation of the current in a series resonance circuit, or of the impedance of a parallel resonant circuit, as a function of frequency is shown in Fig. 2-16.

Resonant circuits can also give rise to an oscillatory waveform if dc rather than ac is applied to them. For example, the current in a series resonant circuit of the form shown in Fig. 2-17 will show an oscillatory

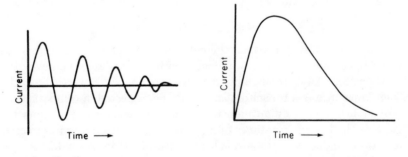

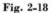
Fig. 2-18
Fig. 2-19

Fig. 2-18 Oscillatory waveform in series resonant circuit when $R^2/4L^2 < 1/LC$.

Fig. 2-19 Buildup and decay of current in a critically damped circuit.

behavior upon closing of the switch S, provided that

$$R^2/4L^2 < 1/LC$$

as shown in Fig. 2-18.
   If

$$R^2/4L^2 = 1/LC$$

the current builds up to a maximum at $t = 2L/R$ sec, and then decays slowly to zero, as shown in Fig. 2-19, and the circuit is called "critically damped." This type of current behavior is made use of in some defibrillators to shape the output pulse. Resonant circuits can also be found in filters, such as bandpass filters, and other applications of medical electronics.

Kirchhoff's Laws

Ohm's law defines the relationship between a voltage across a resistor and a current flowing in that resistor, and is also applicable in its general form to ac, when we deal with impedances rather than resistances. However, it is of only limited value when it is desired to find the relationships between voltages and currents in a complicated network consisting of many inter-related branches. Such networks usually have both nodes and loops. A node is defined as a point where a plurality of currents meet, each current flowing either into or out of the node. A loop is defined as an aggregate of impedances around which a current can flow. Kirchhoff's laws govern the relationships between voltages, currents, loops, and nodes and state that:

1.   The summation of voltages around a loop equals zero.
2.   The summation of currents into a node equals zero.

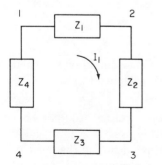

$$\sum V_{12} + V_{23} + V_{34} + V_{41} = 0$$
$$I_1 Z_1 + I_1 Z_2 + I_1 Z_3 + I_1 Z_4 = 0$$

Fig. 2-20   Illustration of Kirchhoff's law pertaining to the summation of voltages. Note: The path from terminal 1 going to terminals 2, 3, 4 and returning again to 1 constitutes a loop.

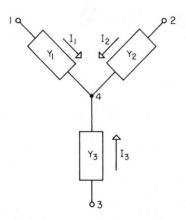

$$\sum I_1 + I_2 + I_3 = 0$$
$$V_{14}Y_1 + V_{24}Y_2 + V_{43}Y_3 = 0$$

Fig. 2-21 Illustration of Kirchhoff's law pertaining to the summation of currents. Y is the admittance of the respective branches. Note: Terminal 4 is a node, a point into which and from which several currents flow.

The application of these laws is very useful in solving for currents and voltages in a network. The law governing the summation of voltages is illustrated in Fig. 2-20. The law governing the summation of currents into a node is illustrated in Fig. 2-21.

An example that specifically works out these relationships is given in Appendix C and deals with a frequently encountered network configuration commonly referred to as the Wheatstone bridge.

Either of Kirchhoff's laws can be used for calculating unknown currents or voltages in a network; the choice of the method will depend on which one yields fewer unknowns and therefore fewer equations.

Network Theorems

The following network theorems are useful in simplifying calculations in networks that would otherwise be laborious or difficult to solve; some terms will be illustrated first.

Theorem 1 *Sources* Sources are either voltage sources or current sources. The symbol for a voltage source is usually a circle, adjacent to which there is either a plus sign or an arrow, denoting the polarity of the source; the symbol for a current source is a rectangle with an inscribed arrow; and the symbol for a signal source or waveform is a circle inscribed with a horizontal S. Other signs are sometimes used; any accompanying text usually explains what is meant, if other signs are used.

Theorem 2   Linear Networks   A network is linear if a change in voltage produces a corresponding change in current—e.g., if the voltage is increased by 5%, the current will also be increased by 5%, and vice versa. A network may be linear over the entire range of voltages and currents that may flow in that network, or it may be linear over only part of its range.

Theorem 3   Superposition   The current flowing through any point in any linear network is the sum of all individual currents at that point. Similarly, the potential difference existing between any two points in that network as a result of multiple voltage sources applied simultaneously within the network is the sum of all the individual potential differences that would have arisen between those two points, had the respective voltages acted individually or separately.

Theorem 4   Reciprocity   If a source in a linear network produces a current I in a branch of that network, then the source, when placed in that branch, will produce a current I in the original branch.

Theorem 5   Thévenin's Theorem   Any linear network containing one or more sources of voltage and having two terminals behaves, insofar as any load impedance connected across these terminals is concerned, as though the network and its generators were equivalent to a simple generator having an internal impedance Z and a generated voltage E, where E is the voltage that appears across the terminals when no load impedance is connected and Z is the impedance measured between the terminals when all sources in the network are short-circuited.

Theorems 1–4 are given for reference and will not be further discussed; but it will be helpful to illustrate an application of Thévenin's theorem.

Consider part of a ground monitor shown in Fig. 2-22. What is the voltage and impedance seen by load Z_{L1} which would, for example, be due to a

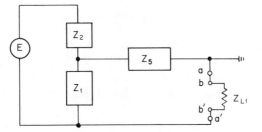

Fig. 2-22   Application of Thévenin's theorem to part of a ground monitor.

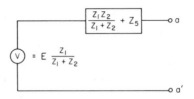

Fig. 2-23 Equivalent circuit of Fig. 2-22 with terminals a–a′ open circuited.

short-circuit? According to Thévenin's theorem, we must (a) find the open circuit voltage across terminals a–a′ with Z_{L1} disconnected and (b) short-circuit voltage source E and find the impedance looking into terminals a–a′.

Under those conditions, the voltage across terminals a–a′ will be given by $EZ_1/(Z_1 + Z_2)$, and the impedance looking into terminals a–a′ will be given by Z_5 in series with Z_1 and Z_2 in parallel, or $[Z_1 \cdot Z_2/(Z_1 + Z_2)] + Z_5$. The equivalent circuit of this configuration is shown in Fig. 2-23.

The application of Thevenin's theorem to a complete ground monitor is discussed in Appendix K.

Filters

Filters are networks that transmit frequencies within one or more frequency bands and attenuate frequencies outside those bands. The most frequently encountered filters are low-pass, high-pass, and bandpass filters.

The most common filters in medical electronics equipment are low-pass filters, which filter out transients—spikes—but permit the passage of signal frequencies. Filters may also add undesirable capacitances to the line, thereby causing additional leakage currents. Two basic filter configurations exist—T sections and Pi sections, shown in Figs. 2-24 and 2-25, respectively. Figures 2-24 and 2-25 show only one section of each type of filter. Several such sections may be cascaded, to make the slope at the cutoff frequency sharper. The cutoff frequency of a filter is defined, in simplified terms, as the frequency above or below which it is no longer possible to transmit information through the filter. For example, it may be desired to pass only a certain band or to reject another band. An example of the latter is the so-called high-pass filter which rejects frequencies below a certain frequency such as, for example, frequencies below 60 Hz, so that they cannot be picked up from the power supply and contaminate whatever

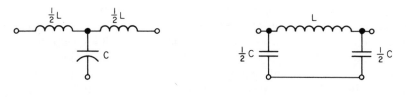

Fig. 2-24 Fig. 2-25

Fig. 2-24 T filter section. $X_L = j\omega L$, $X_C = -j/\omega C$.
Fig. 2-25 Pi filter section. $f_c = 1/\pi(LC)^{1/2}$, where f_c is the nominal cutoff frequency of filter.

information is to be transmited or displayed. An unintended filtering action is sometimes due to the inadequacy of certain components, so that frequencies above or below a certain band cannot be passed.

An example of the latter is the EKG chart recorder. Most chart recorders have a cutoff frequency of 100 Hz, which means that frequencies above 100 Hz are no longer contained in the output of the chart recorder. This is due to the inertia of the recording needle which does in fact act as a filter since it cannot, in most cases, follow frequency variations greater than about 100 Hz. An EKG oscilloscope does not use a recording needle or stylus and therefore provides a much higher frequency response, generally up to about 2,500 Hz. Therefore, even though it is constructed as a so-called dc amplifier for reasons of stability of output, a capacitor is usually used somewhere in the input circuit, and this capacitor limits the low-frequency response of the EKG oscilloscope, so that most EKG oscilloscopes will not pass frequencies below about 0.05 Hz.

In transmitting EKG information by telemetry, filters are frequently used to transmit only desired bands—e.g., 0.05 Hz–200 Hz—to limit the pickup of any extraneous interfering frequencies. For optimum and faithful rendition of information passing through the filter, the delay introduced by the filter, which is inevitable, should be as constant as possible throughout the passband.

The reader who is interested in the topic of filters may refer to the bibliography at the end of this chapter.

Transients and Pulses

Transient waveforms are often thought of in terms of interference—voltage or current spikes that occur as a result of sudden interruption of a current flowing in circuits having inductance, unintentional coupling of circuits, pickup of interference from long wires that act as antennas, and so on. These are undesired transients, and we will be concerned with them when we wish to protect equipment from interference, by adequately shielding such equipment, grounding it properly, and so on. But transients are sometimes deliberately generated for a purpose, in which case they are usually referred to as pulses. The most frequent medical application of such pulses occurs in defibrillators, used to administer an electric shock to patients who have suffered from heart arrest. The energy used in a defibrillator is usually derived from charging one or more capacitors, and discharging the stored energy through a specially designed network. The voltage pulses generated by a defibrillator are of the order of 800–1600 V, and equipment connected to the patient for observation, monitoring, or other purposes must be protected against these voltages, for one cannot assume that such other equipment will be disconnected from the patient when and if he needs to be defibrillated. A more detailed treatment of defibrillators, the waveforms they produce, and the shaping circuits employed to produce these waveforms will be found in Appendix D.

Semiconductors

A. *Diodes*

A semiconductor diode is a device that does not conduct equally well in both directions. The simplest way to visualize a diode is in terms of a switch; when the voltage across its two terminals is applied in one direction the switch is open, and when the direction of voltage is reversed, the switch is closed. The actual characteristics of diodes vary somewhat from these ideal characteristics; actual diode characteristics for a germanium diode are shown in Fig. 2-26.

It will be seen that the diode is a good example of a nonlinear device—i.e., the current through the diode does not increase or decrease proportionately with a corresponding increase or decrease of the applied voltage. In the region of the forward characteristic as shown in Fig. 2-26, the diode does not commence to act as a closed switch until a minimum forward voltage—about 0.2 V in the case of a germanium diode—has been reached. Also, the reverse characteristic of the diode will be seen as a finite, though very large, resistance rather than an open circuit. When the reverse voltage becomes too large, the diode "breaks down," and any further increase in the reverse voltage produces a large amount of reverse current.

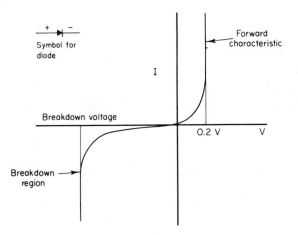

Fig. 2-26   Typical diode characteristics.

Primary uses of diodes in medical electronics equipment occur in power supplies for rectifying alternating current, in current limiters, where they are employed in a back-to-back configuration for protection against current discharges and equipment internal faults, and in many signal-processing circuits.

B.   *Transistors*

Transistors are semiconductor devices with three terminals, used to amplify voltages or currents. The junction transistor, for example, is a current amplifier and has a base, an emitter, and a collector, while the field-effect transistor—FET—has a gate, a source, and a drain and is a device sensitive to voltage variations on its gate. We will be concerned mostly with junction transistors where we distinguish between NPN and PNP transistors. NPN transistors require a positive supply voltage to be applied to the collector terminal, and PNP transistors require a negative supply voltage. The symbol used for the emitter of a transistor of the NPN configuration is an arrow pointing away from the base, indicating that its collector is to be supplied with a positive supply voltage; an arrow pointing toward the base is used in a transistor employing the PNP configuration, indicating that its collector requires a negative supply voltage. These two configurations are shown in Figs. 2-27 and 2-28, respectively.

A signal current flows into the base of the transistor and is amplified, causing a larger current to flow in the load resistor R_L in the collector circuit, connected between the collector and the supply voltage. The re-

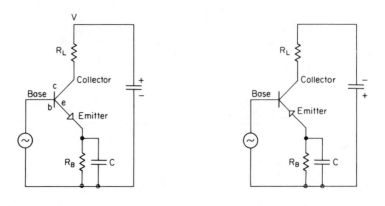

Fig. 2-27   Fig. 2-28

Fig. 2-27   Transistor in NPN configuration.
Fig. 2-28   Transistor in PNP configuration.

sistor R_B and capacitor C serve to bias the base with respect to the emitter; both Figs. 2-28 and 2-29 show a transistor circuit in the so-called common-emitter configuration. Typical output characteristics of an NPN transistor with both varying base currents and varying collector-to-emitter voltages are shown in Fig. 2-29.

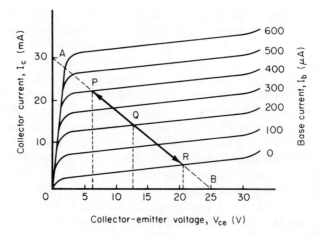

Fig. 2-29   Typical output characteristics of an NPN transistor in the common-emitter configuration.

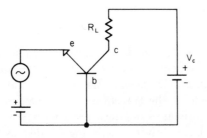

Fig. 2-30 NPN transistor in the common-base configuration.

Another transistor configuration is the common-base configuration, also used for current amplification, and shown for an NPN transistor in Fig. 2-30. Note that for this configuration the emitter must be suitably biased with respect to the base, i.e., a separate bias must be introduced between emitter and base to prevent excessive collector current. The dc gain characteristics of an NPN transistor are discussed in Appendix L.

The third possible configuration is that of the common collector, shown in Fig. 2-31. The common-collector configuration is primarily used for isolation of circuits, since it does not provide any current amplification. The most important factor in transistor technology relates to the ability of the transistor to amplify a current. When currents are relatively small, the transistor can be considered a linear amplifier, and for this reason a small signal current amplification factor has been introduced and designated as h_{fe} or β, denoting the change in collector current for a given change in the base current. A commonly used value of h_{fe} in the common-emitter configuration is of the order of 50.

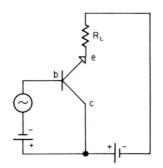

Fig. 2-31 NPN transistor in common-collector configuration.

Transformers

Transformers are used to isolate circuits, and also to step ac voltages up or down; autotransformers perform only the latter function, but do not isolate circuits. Figure 2-32 shows a transformer, and Fig. 2-33 an autotransformer. The side of the transformer to which the voltage source is applied is called the primary side, the other side the secondary. The secondary side may either have both terminals ungrounded, as shown in Fig. 2-32, or one side grounded, as shown in Fig. 2-33. The ratio of the number of turns on the primary side to the number of turns of the secondary side determines whether the transformer acts as a step-up or step-down transformer. Thus, if N_1/N_2 is the primary-to-secondary turns ratio, then the secondary voltage will be $V(N_2/N_1)$, where V is the primary voltage.

When the secondary winding is loaded by a resistance R_s, the resistance seen by the primary circuit becomes

$$(N_1/N_2)^2 R_s = R_{eq\ p}$$

where $R_{eq\ p}$ is the equivalent primary resistance.

In medical electronic equipment, transformers are used in power supplies and in applications where it is desirable to isolate circuits—for example, as their name implies, in isolation transformers.

Difference Amplifier and Common-Mode Rejection

Sometimes the need arises to amplify the difference of two signals, rather than to amplify a single signal. To obtain, for example, a patient's heartbeat, the difference in potential between at least two points on his body

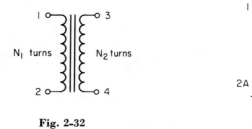

Fig. 2-32 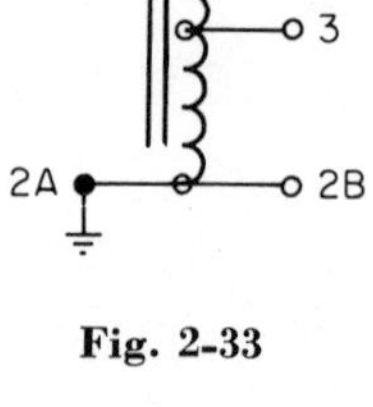   **Fig. 2-33**

Fig. 2-32   Transformer.
Fig. 2-33   Autotransformer.

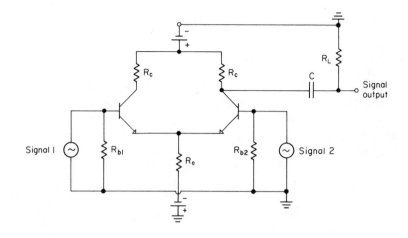

Fig. 2-34 Typical difference amplifier.

must be amplified and neither point should be grounded; both leads are therefore "floating" with respect to ground. To cope with this situation, a difference amplifier having two separate unbalanced amplifier stages* is used, one lead being connected to the input of one amplifier stage, the second lead to the input of the other. A typical difference amplifier is illustrated in Fig. 2-34.

The difference amplifier is so constructed that equal signal inputs from both leads produce no resultant output, while any difference between the signals is amplified. This is an obvious advantage, for any hum (undesired 60-Hz current) picked up in both leads equally will not be amplified, while a difference signal will be.

In practice, a difference amplifier is not perfect; if both input signals are exactly equal, a small amount of the signal that is common to both leads may still be amplified because of imperfections in the difference amplifier. The undesirable amplification of a signal present in both leads is termed "the common-mode gain," and the desirable amplification of the difference between the signals on the two leads is termed the "differential-mode gain." A figure of merit for a difference amplifier is the ratio of the differential gain to the common-mode gain termed the "common-mode rejection ratio." Obviously, the common-mode rejection ratio should be as high as possible; in practice, it is usually 100 or greater.

---

* An unbalanced amplifier has one input and one output terminal effectively grounded.

Telemetry

Everybody is familiar with radio and TV, but perhaps not everybody is familiar with the basic principles of how radio and TV operate. Both employ the principles of modulating a carrier wave with intelligence to produce audio or an image: transmitting the modulated carrier over a distance, receiving and demodulating that carrier, and re-creating the original intelligence. These principles are also used in telemetering the heartbeats of patients by radio to a remote receiver, and in optical isolation systems where EKG information is transmitted by means of a modulated light beam instead of a radio wave. Such telemetry systems completely isolate the patient from the hospital electrical system and therefore from any potentially hazardous currents due to that system.

A radio telemetry system consists of a transmitter and a receiver. The transmitter accepts the information fed to it from a sensor or transducer, modulates that information on a radio-frequency carrier, and feeds the modulated carrier to the antenna of the telemetry transmitter from which it is radiated into space. The antenna of the telemetry receiver picks up the radiated information which is amplified and demodulated; signals similar to the signals that were originally fed to the transmitter result and constitute the output of the telemetry receiver. The principles underlying the remote transmission of heartbeats and consequent isolation of the patient from the hospital electrical system are treated in more detail in Appendix D.

Bibliography

General

Adams, J. E., "Electrical Principles and Practices." McGraw-Hill, New York, 1973.
Alley, C. A., and Atwood, K. W., "Electronic Engineering." Wiley, New York, 1967.
Buban, P., and Schmitt, M., "Understanding Electronics." McGraw-Hill, New York, 1969.
Desoer, C. A., and Kuh E. X., "Basic Circuit Theory." McGraw-Hill, New York, 1969.
Driscoll, F. F., "Analysis of Electric Circuits." Prentice-Hall, Englewood Cliffs, New Jersey, 1973.
Gray, A., and Wallace, G. A., "Principles and Practice of Electrical Engineering." McGraw-Hill, New York, 1962.
Fitzgerald, A. E., Higginbotham, D. E., and Grabel, A., "Basic Electrical Engineering." McGraw-Hill, New York, 1967.
Hagan, W. K., Defibrillation techniques, *Med. Electron. News Data* (July/Aug. 1972).

Hibbs, N., "Basic Electronic Circuits Simplified." Tab Books, 1972.
Howard Sams & Co. Inc., "Reference Data for Radio Engineers." Compiled by ITT contributors, 1972.
Jackson, H. W., "Introduction to Electric Circuits." Prentice-Hall, Englewood Cliffs, New Jersey, 1970.
Leach, D. P., "Basic Electric Circuits." Wiley, New York, 1969.
Liser, E. C., "Electric Circuits and Machines." McGraw-Hill, New York, 1960.
Marion, J. B., "Physical Science in the Modern World." Academic Press, New York, 1974.
Menning, L. A., "Electrical Circuits." McGraw-Hill, New York, 1966.
Novak, Wm., and McPartland, J. F., "Practical Electricity." McGraw Hill, New York, 1964.
McPartland, J. F., and Novak, W., "Electrical Equipment Manual." McGraw-Hill, New York, 1965.
Richter, H. P., "Practical Electrical Wiring." McGraw-Hill, New York, 1972.
Schilling D. L., and Belove, C., "Electronic Circuits: Discrete and Integrated." McGraw-Hill, New York, 1968.
Shillig, H. H., "Electrical Engineering Circuits." Wiley, New York, 1965.
Siskind, C. S., "Electricity, Direct and Alternating Currents." McGraw-Hill, New York, 1955.
Shrader, R. L., "Electrical Fundamentals for Technicians." McGraw-Hill, New York, 1969.
Shore, B. H., "The New Electronics." McGraw-Hill, New York, 1973.
Terman, F. E., "Radio Engineers Handbook." McGraw-Hill, New York, 1955.
Toro, V. C., "Electrical Engineering Fundamentals—Circuit Theory." Prentice-Hall, Englewood Cliffs, New Jersey, 1972.
Weedy, B. M., "Electric Power Systems." Wiley, New York, 1972.
Yanof, M., "Biomedical Electronics." Davis, Philadelphia, Pennsylvania, 1972.

Filters

Anderson, B. D., and Vongpanitlert, S., "Network Analysis and Synthesis." McGraw-Hill, New York, 1973.
Guillemin, E. A., "Synthesis of Passive Networks." Wiley, New York, 1962.
Kuo, F. F., "Network Analysis and Synthesis." Wiley, New York, 1966.

Transformers

Grossner, N. R., "Transformers for Electronic Circuits." McGraw-Hill, New York, 1967.

Telemetry

Gruenberg, E. L. (Editor-in-Chief), "Handbook of Telemetry and Remote Control." McGraw-Hill, New York, 1967.
Stiltz, H. L., "Aerospace Telemetry." Prentice-Hall, Englewood Cliffs, New Jersey, 1964.

Chapter 3

THE ELECTRICAL ENVIRONMENT
OF THE PATIENT

Electricity is used more widely today than ever before. It has had a tremendous impact on our lives and has brought us many benefits. In the field of medicine, numerous advances in diagnosis and treatment have been made as a result of its use and application. Yet, its ability to do good is also accompanied by its potential for doing harm.

In hospitals, the danger of explosions in operating rooms using flammable anesthetics has long been recognized. Elaborate precautions for the prevention of sparking were instituted long ago and are routinely taken today to minimize this hazard. Some other dangers relate to electric shock. Human beings are known to be endangered when they contact live wires carrying voltages of sufficient magnitude for harm. But, until recently, safety precautions against electric shock have not addressed themselves specifically to the hospital environment, the basic protection needs having been assumed to be similar both outside and within the hospital. However, with the advent of implanted devices and electronic diagnostic equipment, new and additional dangers have been recognized because the use of such equipment on a patient can make him sensitive to much smaller electric currents than before. The precautions historically taken against electric shock are therefore no longer adequate in today's hospital environment. Much of the succeeding discussion will address itself to providing the necessary improvements in safety levels to overcome these new hazards.

The response by humans to electric currents has been investigated for some time. Projections from experiments conducted on animals have been made, but the applicability of these results to humans is not known with certainty. There is general agreement, however, as to the levels of current required to produce given reactions in humans. These current levels are given in Table 3-1; they apply to adults subjected to ac currents at the power-line frequencies of 60 Hz. This table deals primarily with the *external* application of electric power to the humans but, for comparison, also shows the effects of internal application at less than 1 mA.

Body Resistance

To electric currents, the human body represents a resistance to current flow between the points of entry and exit. If this resistance were constant, a progressively larger voltage applied across the two points of contact would cause a proportional increase of current flow through the body. At some value of voltage, the current flow would be large enough to have the effects indicated in Table 3-1. Although the assumption of constant resistance permits an appreciation to be gained of the role of voltage in electric shock, it is not an adequate representation of the electrical behavior of the body. Body resistance is not constant; it varies considerably. For fixed entry and exit points, the degree of contact, for example, and skin moisture affect resistance considerably. And, considering all the possible ways by which electrodes can come into contact with the body, body resistance can take on a large variety of different values. For example, a dry hand grip often has a resistance as high as 1 megohm, whereas a similar grip with wet hands may exhibit a resistance smaller than 1000 ohms. Chemical action can also take place that will change the resistance between two points as the voltage is increased. Hence, body resistance is a rather complex quantity and is not very predictable; it is therefore very difficult to predict the current flow in humans in any given situation.

The type of electric power also causes varying body reactions. When that power provides ac, the impedance of the body will not necessarily

Table 3-1
Effect of 60-Hz AC Currents on Adult Humans

Less than 1 mA	Imperceptible when externally applied; through myocardium can induce ventricular fibrillations down to 20 μA.
1–10 mA	Mild to painful sensation.
More than 10 mA	If contacted by hand or arm, may paralyze this region and cause inability to release grip.
More than 30 mA	Breathing frequently stops.
75–250 mA	Causes ventricular fibrillation.
More than 4 amp	Paralyzes the heart.
More than 5 amp	Causes burning of tissues.

equal the dc resistance in magnitude. The frequency of the ac has a pro-
nounced effect upon the current path taken within the body between entry
and exit points. At low frequencies, such as are used in power lines, current
flows in a manner similar to direct current. It distributes itself throughout
the body and may interfere with normal body functions. Table 3-1 applies
to these frequencies. At high frequencies, current tends to travel along the
extreme outside surfaces and therefore interferes less with body functions.
This current concentration along outer surfaces, however, makes burning of
skin more likely. The borderline between low and high frequencies is near
10 kHz.

It has been indicated that body reaction correlates closely with the
quantity of current applied. Recalling that current results from the application of voltage to a resistance (or impedance), these two factors thus are
crucial to current control. Not much can be done to control body resistance.
Hence, the control over excessive current lies in limiting the voltages
accessible across the patient under all conditions.

When electrodes are internally applied, the body resistance is often
lowered to within the 200–1000-ohm region. For a given voltage, current
can then flow much more readily than when the voltage is applied externally. Furthermore, current then frequently flows near the heart region,
where it can interfere with its normal rhythm. When current reaches a
sufficiently large magnitude, ventricular fibrillation can result. Unfortunately, it takes very little current to cause a serious hazard, the quantity
having been found in animals to be as small as 20 μA. This type of electric
shock is known as microshock.

This magnitude of current is often encountered in our normal living
environment and is usually harmless. For example, in the average home,
common appliances are permitted to have a leakage current up to 5 mA
(5000 μA) from the internal mechanisms to the outer case. When we use
these appliances, connected to a power receptacle by means of a two-
prong plug (rather than the more recent 3-prong versions), we are often
exposed to such a leakage current and we seldom even notice its presence.
This current flows into ground somewhere in our homes, yet is of sufficient
magnitude that it would endanger a person with implanted devices if that
person were to be located somewhere along the flow path of the current.
Unless proper and very special precautions are therefore taken in a hospital,
such a current, generated anywhere in the hospital, might flow along
some metallic path near enough to the patient to cause the patient to be
exposed to a hazardous voltage level.

Special precautions to prevent microshock fall into two broad categories:
application of improved grounding systems, and isolation techniques. In
general, the safety precautions are designed around a patient whose body

resistance is assumed to be 500 ohms, which value has been standardized for convenience but is consistent with the range of resistance normally experienced in patients with implanted devices. The presently assumed safe value of current is 10 μA. Taken together, these values mean that a voltage applied to a patient must not exceed

$$V = IR = 10 \times 500 = 5000\,\mu V = 5\,mV$$

This value has been adopted by the National Fire Protection Association (NFPA) as the objective for facilities where implanted devices are in use.

Single-Point Grounds

The basic patient-protection problem against remotely located faults is depicted in Fig. 3-1, which shows two rooms of a building in which a

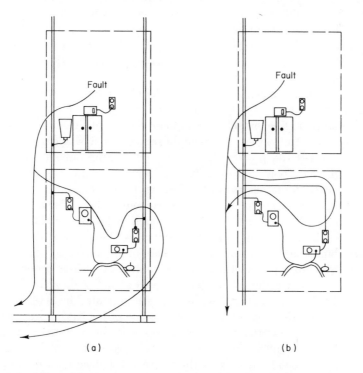

(a)   (b)

Fig. 3-1. Effect of fault currents from other locations. A fault in another room causes fault-current flow through the patient because equipment in the patient's room is (a) grounded to different house grounds and (b) grounded at different locations along a single house ground.

patient with implanted devices or instruments is located. If a fault occurs in an equipment located in a room other than the patient's, a ground current may develop that flows back to earth ground. The paths taken by this current may be numerous and may well include a path through the patient, despite the fact that the patient is located quite remotely from the source of trouble. The currents may not even be due to faults but could be leakage currents from equipments well within permissible limits. In Fig. 3-1a, the two instruments connected to the patient are grounded via the third U-ground conductor in the power cord. Each receptacle, however, is grounded to a different house ground, in this example a water pipe. The current from the fault divides in such a way that a portion of the fault current travels via each instrument and the patient leads to house ground. Suppose that, after recognizing that two different ground pipes can cause this hazard, one connects the grounds from all the receptacles to the same pipe. This connection is shown in Fig. 3-1b, which also reveals its shortcoming. Even though both receptacles are tied to the same pipe, their attachment at different locations permits a portion of the fault current still to enter the patient area. Since fault currents are not quantitatively known and predictable, the voltage between the attachment points may still be larger than the safe limits. This arrangement, therefore, is not adequate.

A further improvement consists of tying all grounds within the patient room to one point on this pipe, as shown in Fig. 3-2. With this change, any fault originating outside the patient room can no longer have any influence upon the patient. The establishment of a single-point ground therefore solves the problem of hazards originating outside the patient room. But what about faults originating within the patient room? Suppose a fault occurs in one instrument, as shown in Fig. 3-2b. A possible fault current will enter the ground of the instrument and could divide into two paths. One path leads back via the U-ground of the power plug. But the other leads through the patient, where it may well be of sufficient magnitude to harm him. Further precautions are therefore required. In Fig. 3-2c, the instrument utilizes patient leads that are well isolated from ground. Thus, the current flow via the two paths is altered so that only a small percentage of the fault current passes through the patient. The actual amount of current depends upon the degree of isolation of the patient lead and the seriousness of the fault. With proper equipment design, this isolation can usually be made sufficiently large that fault currents are, for practical purposes, precluded from entering the patient. Not all equipment, however, can be isolated. If we consider again Fig. 3-2, the use of isolated patient leads would provide added protection. However, the possibility of having outside currents entering a patient locale must be avoided in any case,

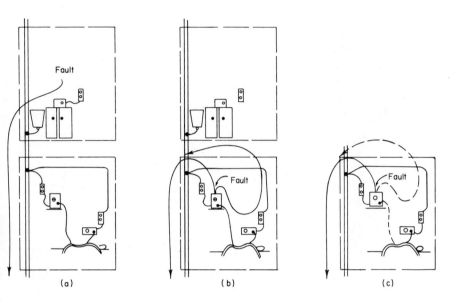

Fig. 3-2. Single-point ground in patient room (a) protects patient from fault currents originating outside his room but (b) not from those originating in his room; isolated patient leads (c) help protect from the latter.

because current magnitudes are totally uncontrolled. One can never know when a safe facility has been achieved under such conditions.

Ground Equalization

To cope with the potential hazards originating within the locale, all the ground points that might be in contact with the patient must be tied together by means of a low-impedance path. This procedure is known as ground equalization. Consider again Fig. 3-2. The two current paths arise because both points are not strapped together. A current travels along each path, the magnitudes being determined by the resistances of the paths. At the same time, the patient is exposed to the voltage drop due to the entire path. This situation is avoided when the two grounds are tied together, as in Fig. 3-3. Now, the voltage drop is drastically reduced, and the patient is exposed to only the small remaining voltage drop across the ground-equalization bus. The resistance of the bus becomes a bypass to the patient for electric currents. How effectively the bus bypasses all potential hazardous currents will depend upon how small the bus resistance

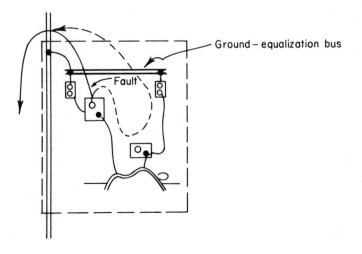

Fig. 3-3.   Ground equalization tends to keep voltage drops among grounds within a room small even in the event of fault.

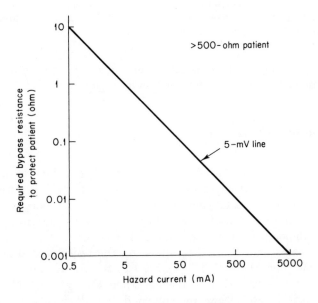

Fig. 3-4.   Effectiveness of patient-ground bypass. Protection against larger currents requires a smaller total resistance in the bypass. Practical ground wiring cannot easily be kept under 0.1 ohm, thus limiting the effectiveness of ground wires to hazards under 50 mA.

is made. The division of current between patient and bus is inversely proportional to the resistance of each, as illustrated in Fig. 3-4. A patient resistance of 500 ohms is assumed. The curve shows how much ground current may flow before the patient-voltage limit of 5 mV has been reached, as the ground equalization resistance is varied. In practice, it is difficult to keep the bus resistance values, including connections, under 0.1 ohm. This value, however, effectively limits fault currents to less than 50 mA.

Ground equalization is the most effective means for protecting patients against microshock due to sources within the locale. It minimizes the consequences of leakage but does not prevent any leakage from occurring. It does not, therefore, obviate the need to ensure that current leakage from equipments in use within the installation is small and that the equipment is otherwise safe.

Isolated Power Systems

In conventional power-distribution systems, one of the power lines is tied to earth ground. When some fault occurs, current will flow via ground back to the power source. In an isolated power system, a transformer is placed between the power source and the instrument load. Whereas the transformer input can have one of its power leads grounded, none of its output power leads are tied to earth ground. A high-impedance path from the isolated power lines to ground still exists, however, due to winding capacitance, transformer leakage, and monitoring devices. When a fault develops from one of the isolated power lines to ground, the amount of current flowing in the ground will be much smaller than it would be in a conventionally grounded power system. This is so because the high-impedance path reduces current flow.

Isolated power systems are used where flammable anesthetics are employed. In that connection, the reduced current flow for a given fault tends to prevent the development of electric arcing. Such isolated power systems require, by NFPA regulation, monitoring devices that sense ground current and provide warnings and alarms when specific current limits are exceeded. Unfortunately, practical designs in present-day use have alarm settings at current levels above those ensuring microshock protection, and they seldom shut off power when thresholds have been exceeded. Furthermore, the monitoring devices can actually introduce a small ground current of their own into the system. Thus isolated power systems do not present a particularly favorable environment for microshock protection. However, such facilities can be made safe against microshock by the additional installation of single-point grounds and ground equalization.

Bibliography

Aitkulova, A. U., On the Relative Danger of Direct and Alternating Currents, *Trudi Konf. Elektrotravme, Frunze, Soviet Union.* Kirgiz Acad. Sci. Publ. House, 1957.

Azhibayev, K. A., On the Question of the Relative Danger of Direct and Alternating Currents, *Trudi Konf. Elektrotravme, Frunze, Soviet Union.* Kirgiz Acad. Sci. Publ. House, 1957.

Barry, W. F., Jr., Starmer, C. F., Whalen, R. E., and McIntosh, H. D., Electric Shock Hazards in Radiology Departments, *Amer. J. Roentg.* 95 (1965).

Bibliography of Electric Shock Hazards in the Hospital Environment, Univ. of British Columbia.

Bibliography on Electrical Hazards, Safety and Standards in Biomedical Engineering. Beckman Instrum. Inc., Fullerton, California.

Carlson, A. J., Comparative Physiology of the Invertebrate Heart. VI. The Excitability of the Heart During the Different Phases of the Heart Beat, *Amer. J. Physiol.* 16 (1906).

Carlson, A. J., On the Mechanism of the Refractory Period in the Heart, *Amer. J. Physiol.* 18 (1907).

Dalziel, C. F., The Effects of Electric Shock on Man, *Safety Fire Protect. Tech. Bull.* 7, U.S. At. Energy Comm. Washington, D.C. (1956).

Dalziel, C. F., Threshold 60-Cycle Fibrillating Currents, *AIEE Trans. Power Appl. Syst.* 79 (Oct. 1960).

Dalziel, C. F., and Lee, W. R., Reevaluation of Lethal Electric Currents, *IEEE Trans. Inst. Gen. Appl.* IGA-4, No. 5 (Sept. 1968).

Dalziel, C. F., Electric Shock Hazard, *IEEE Spectrum* 9, No. 2 (1972).

Dobbie, A. K., Electricity in Hospitals, *Biomed. Eng. (GB)* 7, No. 1 (1972).

Electricity: A Subtle Menace in Hospitals, *Sci. Dim. (Canada)* 3, No. 1 (Feb. 1971).

Ellerbe, Report on Electrical Hazards within Medical Facilities, Ellerbe Architects, St. Paul, Minnesota.

Epidemiological Notes: Deaths from Electric Current, *Publ. Health Rep. U.S. Dept. HEW.* 75, 962 (1960).

Ferris, L. P., King, B. G., Spence, R. W., and Williams, H. B., Effects of Electric Shock on the Heart, *Elet. Eng.* 55, (May 1936).

Friedlander, G. D., Electricity in Hospitals: Elimination of Lethal Hazards, *IEEE Spectrum* 8, No. 9 (Sept. 1971).

Han, J., Millet, D., Chizzonitti, B., and Moe, G. K., Temporal Dispersion of Recovery of Excitability in Atrium and Ventricle as a Function of Heart Rate, *Amer. Heart J.* 71 (Apr. 1966).

Han, J., Garcia de Jalon, P. D., and Moe, G. K., Fibrillation Threshold of Premature Ventricular Responses, *Circ. Res.* 18 (1966).

Hooker, D. R., On Recovery of the Heart in Electric Shock, *Amer. J. Physiol.* 91 (1929).

Hooker, D. R., Kouwenhoven, W. B., and Langworthy, O. R., The Effects of Alternating Electrical Currents on the Heart, *Amer. J. Physiol.* 103, 444 (1933).

Hopps, J. A., and Roy, O. Z., Electrical Hazards in Cardiac Diagnosis and Treatment, *Med. Electron. Biol. Eng.* **1** (1963).

Hopps, J. A., Shock Hazards in the Operating Rooms and Patient Care Areas, *Anesthesiology* (Jan. 1969).

Hughes, J. P. W., Emergencies in General Practice: Electric Shock and Associated Accidents, *Brit. Med J.* **1** (Apr. 1956).

Kantrowitz, P., Electrical Safety in Hospitals, *Instrum. Technol.* **19**, No. 8 (Aug. 1972).

King, B. G., The Effect of Electric Shock on Heart Action with Special Reference to Varying Susceptibility in Different Parts of the Cardiac Cycle, Columbia Univ. Thesis, Aberdeen Press, New York, 1934.

Kiselev, A. P., Threshold Value of Safe Currents of Commercial Frequency *Vop. Elektoborud. Elekt-snabsh. Elekt. Izmerenii. Sob. MITT* **17** (1963).

Kline, R. L., and Friauf, J. B., "Electric Shock, its Causes and Prevention," NAV-SHIPS 250-660-42. U.S. Govt. Printing Office, Washington, D.C. (1954).

Knickerbocker, G. G., Fibrillating Parameters of Direct and Alternating (20 Hz) Currents Separately and in Combination—An Experimental Study, *IEEE Trans. Commun.* **COM-21**, No. 9 (Sept. 1973).

Kouwenhoven, W. B., and Langworthy, O. R., Effect of Electric Shock, *Trans. Amer. Inst. EE* **49** (1930).

Kouwenhoven, W. B., Hooker, D. R., and Lotz, E. L., Electric Shock Effect of Frequency, *Elect. Eng.* **55** (Apr. 1936).

Kouwenhoven, W. B., Knickerbocker, G. G., Chestnut, R. W., Milnor, W. R., and Sass, D. J., AC Shocks of Varying Parameters Affecting the Heart, *AIEE Trans. Comm. Elect.* **78** (May 1959).

Langworthy, O. R., and Kouwenhoven, W. B., What are the Effects of Electric Shock, *Elect. Eng.* **50** (1931).

Lee, W. R., The Nature and Management of Electric Shock, *Brit. J. Anesth.* **36**, 572 (1964).

Lee, W. R., Deaths from Electric Shock in 1962 and 1963, *Brit. Med. J.* **2** (Sept. 1965).

Leeming, M. N., Ray, C., and Howland, W. S., Low Voltage, Direct Current Burns, *J. Amer. Med. Ass.* **214**, No. 9 (Nov. 1970).

Levy, M. J., and Lillehei, C. W., Apparatus, Application and Indications for Fibrillatory Cardiac Arrest, *Surgery* **53** (Feb. 1963).

Lown, B., Newman, J., Amarasingham, R., Berkovits, B. V., Comparison of Alternating Current with Direct Current Electroshock across Closed Chest, *Amer. J. Cardiol.* **10**, 223 (1962).

Lown, B., Perlroth, M. G., Kaidbey, S., Abe, T., and Harken, D. E., Cardioversion of Atrial Fibrillation, *New England J. Med.* **269**, 325 (1963).

Noordijk, J. A., Oey, F. T. I., and Tebra, W., Myocardial Electrodes and the Danger of Ventricular Fibrillation, *Lancet* **1**, 975 (1961).

Osypka, P., Problems of Safety in the Use of Electromedical Apparatus on Human Beings, *Bull. Ass. Suisse Elect.* (Switz. in German) **63**, No. 19 (Sept. 1972).

Peleska, B., Optimal Parameters of Electrical Impulses for Defibrillation by Condenser Discharges, *Circ. Res.* **18** (1966).

Pengelly, L. D., and Klassen, G. A., Myocardial Electrodes and the Danger of Ventricular Fibrillation, *Lancet* (June 3, 1961).

Prevost, J. L., and Battelli, F., Death by Electric Currents, Alternating Current at Low Voltage, *J. Physiol. Pathol. Gen.* **1** (1899).

Prevost, J. L., and Battelli, F., Death by Electric Currents, Direct Current, *J. Physiol. Pathol. Gen.* **2** (1900).

Starmer, C. F., Whalen, R. E., and McIntosh, H. D., Hazards of Electrical Shock in Cardiology, *Amer. J. Cardiol.* **14** (Oct. 1964).

Sugimoto, T., Schaal, S. F., and Wallace, A. G., Factors Determining Vulnerability to Ventricular Fibrillation Induced by 60-CPS Alternating Current, *Circ. Res.* **21** (1967).

Walter, C. W., Electrical Hazards in Hospitals. Nat. Acad. Sci. (1970).

Wegria, R., and Wiggers, C. J., Factors Determining the Production of Ventricular Fibrillation by Direct Current (With Note on Chronaxie), *Amer. J. Physiol.* **131** (1940).

Wegria, R., and Wiggers, C. J., Production of Ventricular Fibrillation by Alternating Currents, *Amer. J. Physiol.* **131** (1940).

Weinberg, D. I., Artley, J. L., Whalen, R. E., and McIntosh, H. D., Electric Shock Hazards in Cardiac Catheterization *Circ. Res.* **11** (1962).

Wiggers, C. J., Studies of Ventricular Fibrillation Caused by Electric Shock; Cinematographic and Electrocardiographic Observation of the Natural Process in the Dog's Heart; Its Inhibition by Potassium and the Revival of Coordinated Beats by Calcium, *Amer. Heart J.* **5** (1930).

Williams, H. B., King, B. G., Ferris, L. P., and Spence, P. W., Susceptibility of the Heart to Electric Shock in Different Phases of the Cardiac Cycle, *Proc. Soc. Exp. Biol. Med.* **31** (1934).

Chapter 4

THE CHARACTERISTICS OF INSTALLATIONS

The medical practitioner is assisted in the performance of his activities by a host of diagnostic and therapeutic instruments that are intended to enhance his ability to be of service to his patient. These instruments must be capable of furnishing information reliably in the sense that the physician must be able fully to trust the information provided by the equipment. Incorrect or erratic information could lead to faulty diagnosis or treatment and might thereby constitute a serious hazard. In addition, the mere use of the equipment, somehow interconnected with other devices, can introduce extraneous hazards to patients, usually electrical in nature, which may complicate the patient's original condition or might expose him to new health hazards. It is therefore very important that the causes of these potential hazards be fully understood and that the necessary steps be taken to preclude their presence.

An instrument may supply erroneous information because it is improperly designed or calibrated, or because it may be improperly connected. On the other hand, the facility might have been inadequately wired or the instruments improperly installed. The grounding system plays the major role in the latter. If all equipments could be installed in a fixed location and were never moved, a safe installation could be more readily achieved than in the more practical situation where instruments are frequently relocated and are often disconnected and reconnected. Maintaining a safe installation under these conditions requires conscious adherence to sound safety principles and frequent safety checking.

The patient, of course, is not the only one to be protected; the doctor and other hospital personnel are also exposed to similar hazards. The degree of safety obtainable is always cost-related. This, as well as our inability to predict all safety hazards in advance, precludes the establishment of one fixed set of safety rules throughout the health-care facility. Instead, the degree of protection is made dependent upon the seriousness of the consequences to be expected, i.e., the degree to which life and health might be jeopardized. A given hazard condition might well be dangerous to humans only under some specific circumstances. A minute electric current, for example, may cause serious injury to a person via an implanted device, whereas the very same current will be totally harmless when applied to the outer skin of some other person.

The concept of having more stringent safety protection for unusual hazards is not new. In hospitals, safety requirements usually fall into three categories: protection of patients with implanted devices or exposed interiors, protection of power sources for essential functions from accidental interruption, and protection from explosion hazards. The most stringent safety requirements are applied only in very specific locations, such as in operating rooms. As long as the activities that might entail an unusual hazard are confined to those parts of the facility in which the stringent safety protection is furnished, safety can be reasonably assured. But under some circumstances, certain activities—for example, treatment in connection with implantable devices or care of patients who use an embedded catheter—may have to take place elsewhere, as is the case when a part of a hospital is filled to capacity. Unless additional steps are then taken to protect such patients, they may be unnecessarily exposed to new hazards.

Microshock Protection

A patient wearing an implanted device or a patient with an inserted catheter may be vulnerable to the adverse effects of even small electric currents, since these currents under such circumstances are more readily diverted to electrically sensitive heart muscle and tissues. To protect against this hazard, additional and severe grounding requirements are imposed upon every metallic device within the room. Such facilities are termed "electrically susceptible patient areas," or ESPA's, and safety requirements for these facilities have now been formalized.

Power-Disruption Protection

If the central power fails, it will have a varying impact upon the people within the facility. Whereas it may constitute no more than a temporary inconvenience for most persons in the hospital, the impact may be vital to others, such as those requiring electrical instrumentation for life sustenance or those in surgery. To provide backup power systems for the entire hospital is economically prohibitive. Instead, all those power lines that require continuity when external power fails are separated from the remaining electrical system and are supplied from an auxiliary power source. The arrangement permits power restoration within 10 seconds of main power failure to those areas having such need.

To accomplish this end, the electrical system is divided into branches according to safety priorities. Distinctions are made among "life-safety branches" serving illumination, alerting and alarm equipment, "life-support branches" for ESPA's, and "critical branches" for lighting and receptacles in critical patient areas. The wall receptacles allocated to each branch must, of course, be distinguishable to hospital personnel so that they will be utilized properly and will, in fact, provide the desired protection in case of power failure.

Explosion Protection

Flammable anesthetics in hospital operating rooms constitute a potential explosive hazard. Safety precautions include specially constructed, partially conducting floors, special clothing, unusual grounding requirements, and isolated electric-power distribution systems in which common electrical faults are unlikely to cause sparking. Emphasis is placed on avoiding all conditions under which static electricity can build up to the strength at which sparking might occur and on methods for gradually discharging static voltages present in the room. With the increasing use of nonflammable anesthetics, the safety requirements for explosion protection are beginning to lose their urgency. Some of these requirements, such as the use of partially conducting flooring, are in conflict with the best practices for microshock protection. This poses a dilemma because the same facility, the operating room, may need protection against both hazards. Simultaneous protection against both microshock and explosion hazard may thus not be fully obtainable in these locations. Unlike ESPA requirements, the safety rules relating to flammable anesthetics, because of their long history of use, have been well codified for some time.

The Role of Grounds

Electric power is normally distributed by means of either two or three insulated wires. Ideally, if none of these conductors were to be tied to earth ground, no electric current would flow in the ground. But when, because of a breakdown in the system, one of these wires accidentally touches earth, the region of contact becomes electrified. Currents in the wires do not necessarily increase under these conditions because the return path is lengthy and contains much resistance to current flow. Thus, protective devices sensitive to overcurrents may not be activated, and the persons in the vicinity of the mishap may, unknowingly, be exposed to serious shock hazards for extended periods of time. To avoid this condition, electric-power distribution systems and other electric devices accessible to the public generally have one of the power leads connected to a metallic ground. Then, when an accidental line grounding occurs from an un-grounded conductor, a large fault current flows that can easily be detected by current-monitoring devices. Power can then be automatically interrupted.

When a power line is grounded at only one location, the electric current normally still flows only in the power lines and not in the ground. As a practical matter, however, because of current leakage from equipments and wires as well as failures and anomalies, some current will even then flow in the ground. This results in voltage drops between various points, all of which are grounds, thus making the electric voltage existing at one ground point different from that existing at another.

One refers to a good ground as being one that, relative to all other grounds in a given locale, is very close to and preferably at exactly the same electric voltage. The emphasis is on a specific locale within which this condition must prevail. What the actual voltage is with respect to earth in any other location is of no concern. Crucial to achieving an electrically safe environment is the good ground in that locale, whether it is the operating room, the hospital kitchen, or someone's living room. To obtain the good ground, all metallic points in the locale must be controlled so that they will be at (almost) the same voltage. In the hospital these points include, for example, all the electrical receptacles, equipment surfaces, bed frames, water supply, waste disposal, and piping.

If it were possible to place together all metallic points in a given locale, no voltage could be developed among grounds, as there would only be one ground point. But in practice, grounds are physically separated by varying distances. The establishment of a good ground is then equivalent to arranging the physical layout so that a single-point ground is closely approximated. This involves careful control over the factors that might create differences in voltages among ground points. There are two ways to cope with electric voltages between two points. One consists of avoiding current flow between the two points, as for example, by diverting currents around the locale. This is usually done quite effectively for currents that do not originate in the locale, but is not usually possible for currents originating within the locale such as those due to electrical instruments in use there. Protection is then provided by minimizing rather than eliminating voltage differences among ground points by controlling the conductors lengths and resistances so as to ensure that voltage differences are below acceptable levels. The way in which length and resistance influences voltage drop is shown in Fig. 4-1. The thin wire in Fig. 4-1a has a resistance of 0.5 ohm, for which the stray current of 100 mA at 60 Hz results in a voltage difference of 50 mV. When a wire of larger diameter but equal length is used, the wire resistance is reduced as in Fig. 4-1b. The resultant resistance of 0.1 ohm, even though passing the same current, reduces the voltage difference to 10 mV. The role of wire length is illustrated in Fig. 4-1c, where doubling the wire length doubles the voltage difference between the ground points.

A complicating factor is the behavior of wiring to currents at higher frequencies, generally above 10,000 Hz. The voltage drop is then governed not only by the wire resistance but also by its shape, the curvature of the wire run, and proximity effects of nearby objects. The impedance between

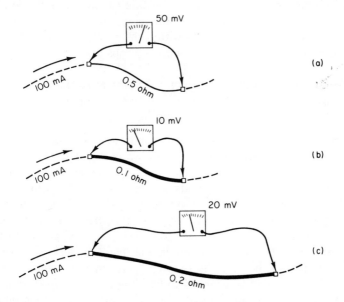

Fig. 4-1 How voltage drop varies with wire size. The heavier lead in (b) reduces the voltage drop over (a) when the same current is flowing in both wires. Doubling the length (c) will double the voltage drop.

points then determines voltage drops. Fortunately, currents at these higher frequencies are less hazardous to humans and play a less significant part in hospital ground safety than those due to power-line frequencies. Wire-resistance considerations therefore usually suffice in determining ground safety.

Grounding in Anesthetizing and ESPA Locations

To ensure proper grounding, the National Fire Protection Association sets forth in a series of publications the methods to be used to establish grounds. These publications describe the detailed steps to be taken to ensure grounding safety in anesthetizing locations and in electrically susceptible patients areas. Although the two requirements differ in some respects, both make extensive use of the principles just outlined. The basic techniques for controlling grounds are the following:

establishment of a single-point ground, as observed from outside the room, by having one single ground connection from the locale to outside points. (Ground currents originating outside cannot enter the locale and therefore cannot cause voltage drops among grounds inside the room.);

control of wire sizes and lengths within the room, to keep voltage drops small, with testing to ensure that voltage drops are below an established limit;

control of the physical layout around the patient so that he is certain to be confined and protected electrically within the ground system of one locale only and has no contact with another.

In an anesthetizing location, all grounds are brought together at a common reference grounding point, as shown in Fig. 4-2. The grounds are subdivided into three ground systems: patient ground, room ground, and the receptacle grounds. All grounds within reach of the patient, such as grounded instrumentation, are connected to the patient ground, while other metallic objects in the room, such as sinks, are connected to the room ground. All plug-in equipments are grounded via the U-ground* of plugs and receptacles. The reference grounding point is located within the electric distribution box for the isolated power system required in anesthetizing locations and is attached to building ground. This establishes a single-point ground leading outside the locale for the patient ground and

---

* The U-ground is the third grounded terminal of a 3-prong plug or receptacle. It gets its name from the shape of the mating pin.

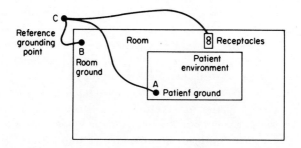

Fig. 4-2 Basic grounding concept for anesthetizing locations. A, patient ground for operating table, anesthesia machine, and other items in contact with patient; B, room ground, for all metallic surfaces near patient and near persons in touch with patient; C, reference grounding point for each electrical power distribution system to which patient ground and room ground are connected.

the reference grounding point. Because of connections to piping, however, it does not constitute a single-point ground for the room ground.

The arrangement for an ESPA is shown in Fig. 4-3. This time, the voltage drops are more closely controlled by direct connection of receptacles into the patient reference grounding bus rather than via the room reference grounding point. With connections to building ground made from the room reference grounding bus, a single-point ground will exist to all points outside of the locale for both patient reference grounding bus and room reference grounding bus.

Under NFPA regulations, any two of points A, B, and C may be combined when feasible in a practical situation. Requirements for both

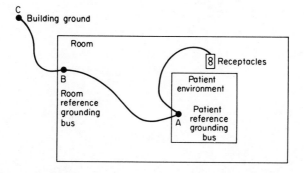

Fig. 4-3 Basic grounding concept for ESPA. A, patient reference grounding bus for all instruments and metallic surfaces that contact patient; B, room reference grounding bus for all other metallic surfaces near patient and near persons in touch with patient; C, building ground to which the ESPA grounding system is joined.

anesthetizing locations and ESPA may then be met simultaneously, as is often necessary in operating rooms. Numerous arrangements are possible within the framework of the NFPA requirements. Two examples are given here. The first, representing a relatively small ESPA, is shown in Fig. 4-4. In this system, the electrical distribution box not only contains the electrical terminals for power and neutral lines but also incorporates the grounding bus (lower portion of box) to which all ground connections within reach of the patient are made. In use, all instruments requiring house power are supplied from the receptacles shown and are grounded via the U-ground conductors carried through the power cords. Other metallic surfaces such as the bed frame must also be grounded, either by a permanent connection to the same ground bus (not shown) or by a grounding lead plugged into the auxiliary ground jack fixture mounted adjacent to the electrical distribution box. The ground bus serves as the patient reference grounding bus and is connected at a single point (the bus itself) to the remaining house grounds. Other patient-ground systems in the same room could also be connected to the same ground bus so that it may serve simultaneously as

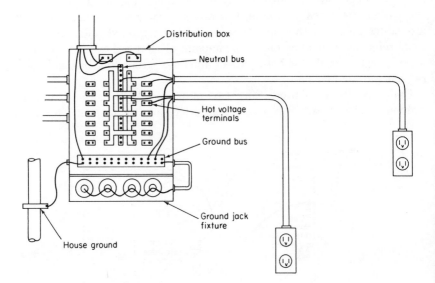

Fig. 4-4 Simple grounding system for electrically susceptible patient area (ESPA). All grounds are tied together at the distribution box. Patient reference and room reference are combined. Instruments are plugged into wall outlets, and all other metallic surfaces within reach of patient are connected to same ground, by permanent wiring or by plugging into ground jacks.

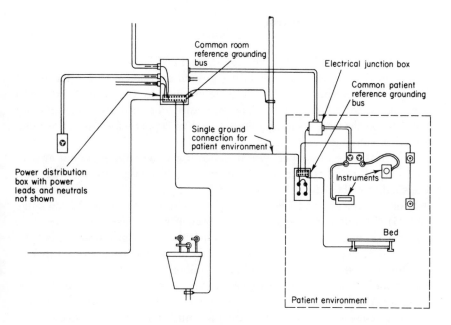

Fig. 4-5 More elaborate grounding system for ESPA showing how patient environment is tied to other grounds with only a single connecting line. Ground leads from electrical receptacles are routed to the patient reference grounding bus.

the room reference grounding bus. This arrangement, although simple, may prove inadequate when the distribution box is not conveniently located near the patient. A more elaborate grounding system may then be necessary, as in Fig. 4-5. The patient environment, shown within the dashed lines, includes a separate grounding bus having fixed screw terminals and several grounding jacks, which represents the patient reference grounding bus for this patient locale. The ground wire carried within each power cord, usually routed with the electric power to the distribution box, is separated and brought back to this grounding bus. An electric junction box is used in practice. Additional grounding jacks may also be located within the patient environment, to make it easier to ground metallic fixtures used in patient care. The important requirement is that all the ground leads within the patient environment terminate at the common patient reference grounding bus. One ground connection is then brought out from this bus to the room reference grounding bus, shown located within the distribution box. This room ground also grounds other metallic surfaces in the room as well as grounds of electrical outlets not associated with the electrically susceptible patient.

Voltage-Drop Control

It was stated earlier that voltage drops must be controlled in order to minimize the influence of circulating ground currents within a locale. At low frequencies, this voltage drop is determined by the path resistance in accordance with Ohm's law. The resistance obtained from one ground point to another is a result of a finite length of copper wire and one or more electrical contacts.

The resistance of copper wire depends upon the cross-sectional area of the conductor and the length of the wire run. The larger the cross section, the smaller will be the resistance per foot of length. This is shown in Table 4-1 for commonly available copper wire, using the American Wire Gauge (AWG) size numbering system. Most branch wiring uses AWG sizes #10, 12, and 14, whereas AWG #16 and 18 may be found in power cords. The interrelationship of wire size, length, and current has been plotted in Fig. 4-6 for a fixed maximum permissible voltage drop of 5 mV. It shows, for example, that for a 10-mA ground current, the run may be as long as 315 ft of AWG #12 copper wire before the 5-mV limit is reached. Although this may suggest that long wire runs are quite safe, the presence of wire connections and their contribution to voltage drop makes it usually necessary to limit wire lengths severely.

Solid copper wire, unless of small diameter, does not bend easily, and

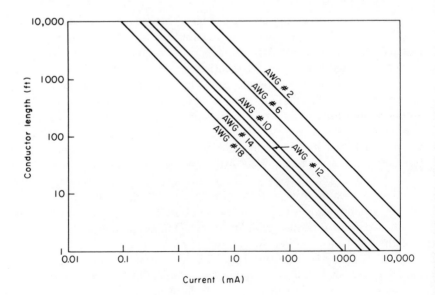

Fig. 4-6   Wire length for 5-mV drop.

Table 4-1
Cross-Sectional Area and Resistance of Copper Wire

Wire size (AWG #)	Cross-sectional area (square inches)	Resistance per foot (milliohms)
000	0.132	0.062
00	0.104	0.078
0	0.083	0.098
2	0.052	0.156
4	0.033	0.249
6	0.021	0.395
8	0.013	0.628
10	0.008	0.999
12	0.005	1.588
14	0.003	2.525
16	0.002	4.016
18	0.001	6.385

to gain greater wire flexibility, stranded wire is often used instead. The latter consists of a number of solid, twisted wire conductors, each having a small diameter. Especially on leads connected temporarily and used with grounding jacks, flexible copper wiring is much to be preferred. The cross-sectional area and the resistance of stranded wire bundles specified by AWG number is approximately equal to that of a solid copper wire with the same AWG number. Sometimes, it may be desired to obtain the added flexibility by connecting several solid conductors in parallel. How the AWG wire size is affected by this procedure is shown in Table 4-2. For example, tying three AWG #18 leads in parallel results in a bundle having the equivalent AWG size 18 minus 4, or AWG #14.

Table 4-2
AWG Size Resulting from Paralleling Conductors

Number of solid conductors in parallel	Subtract from AWG # of each conductor used, to yield AWG # of combination
2	3
3	4
4	5
5	6
6	7
7	8
8	8
9	9

Electrical Contacts

Conductors need to be secured at each end by means of some form of termination. When this connection can be made in a permanent manner, fastening of the conductor is often simply a matter of tightening a screw. A more difficult problem arises in those instances when it is undesirable to make the connection permanent, as in the case of all plugs, jacks, splices, and clips. All temporary connections are notorious for the instability of the resistance value across their surfaces. Voltage drops are unpredictable, making temporary connections a major cause of potentially hazardous grounding situations in health-care facilities. Relatively stable contact resistances are obtained when the outer layers of conductor materials are penetrated and a good contact is made between the inner base materials of both conductors.

A. *The Penetrating Contact*

To achieve a penetrating contact, the outer surfaces of the two wires to be joined are first broken, thus putting the two base-metal surfaces in solid contact with one another. Pressure is most commonly used, either by a screw driver, crimping tool, or other forcing arrangement, but other techniques such as soldering achieve essentially the same result. Good contact over a significant surface area is then obtained over which current flow takes place, and exposure to the atmosphere is avoided over most of the contact surface. Thus, oxidation and corrosion are avoided, and the contact remains secure over long periods of time. The result is a stable contact resistance and a consistent voltage drop across the contact.

The reliability of the connection depends critically upon proper tightening. Any looseness will allow atmospheric action to form a surface film on the conductors that ultimately destroys the effectiveness of the penetrating contact. For example, when using crimping tools, great care must be exercised that a penetrating contact from the exposed wire to the crimping lug is achieved, as well as protection against wire motion; the latter is accomplished by crimping the wire insulation securely to the rear portion of the lug. When the insulation is not properly clamped, the connection from the exposed wire to the lug may loosen in time, thus destroying the effectiveness of the connection.

B. *The Surface-to-Surface Contact*

When two surfaces are brought in contact with one another without benefit of a penetrating contact, the electrical characteristics of the contact depend upon many factors, such as the pressure exerted, the condition of the surfaces, the area of contact, and the surface materials. Instead of the base metals being in contact, the electrical connection is actually made between the surface layers of the two conductors. Among possible surface layers are metal finishes intentionally applied for protection or decorative purposes such as on instrument front panels, and surface layers that result from interaction of the base material with the atmosphere. Often, these surface layers are poor electrical conductors and their depth is not uniform. With time, their characteristics tend to change because of wear or the effects of the atmosphere. Even on a day-to-day basis, the contact resistance across such surfaces is variable and unpredictable. To make things worse, currents flowing across such surfaces tend to modify the characteristics of the surfaces, and when of sufficient magnitude may even cause arcing to take place, which can radically modify the surfaces.

Obviously, surface-to-surface contacts are poor candidates for making reliable connections, but they cannot always be avoided. Plugs and jacks are good examples. The choice of materials plays an important part in maintaining good surface-to-surface contact. Some materials—those forming nonconducting films when exposed to the atmosphere—are particularly bad. Others form conductive films that may not be stable or may be subject to abrasion. Among satisfactory materials are copper and bronze alloys from which electrical plugs are made and gold-plated copper conductors frequently found on multipin connectors. These are applied in conjunction with some spring material used to control contact pressure. This combination is commonly used where a penetrating contact is precluded, but it must be tested frequently to ensure continued electrical integrity.

Regulatory Limitations

In addition to specifying the basic grounding concept, the NFPA also sets limits on wire lengths, resistances, and voltages in anesthetizing and ESPA locations. These regulations are summarized in Table 4-3. Examples of applications of these requirements are presented in Appendix F.

Grounding in Biomedical Instruments

The previous discussion has shown that instruments, plugged into an installation, become a part of the patient grounding system. Because they

Table 4-3
Summary of NFPA Regulations on Lengths and Sizes of Wire, Resistance, and Voltage in Anesthetizing Locations and ESPA[a]

WIRE RUNS

	Maximum length (ft)	Minimum wire size (AWG #)
Anesthetizing locations		
Patient ground		
to reference grounding point	—	10
to remote jacks	15	12
to operating table (when ESPA)	10	10
to anesthesia machine (when ESPA)	10	10
Room ground to reference grounding point	—	10
Metal raceway to panel-board ground	—	12
ESPA		
Patient reference grounding bus		
to room reference grounding bus	—	10
to receptacles	15	12
to patient	5	
to patient bed	5	12
to structure	—	10
Grounding cords	10	10
Metal raceway to panel board	—	12

RESISTANCE

	Maximum resistance (ohms)
Anesthetizing locations	
Ground jacks	0.005
Patient ground to any other ground	0.1
ESPA	
Ground jacks	0.005
Room reference ground bus to any other ground	0.05 at 20 amp
Instruments	
Instrument ground to receptacle U-ground	0.1

VOLTAGE

	Maximum voltage (mV)
Anesthetizing locations or ESPA	
Among grounds around patient	5

[a] These are highlights of key requirements and recommendations. NFPA publications undergo frequent revisions and updating. The latest publications should be consulted for current regulations and all detailed requirements.

can thereby contribute to hazardous ground currents, they must be designed and installed to minimize this possibility.

The grounding system of an instrument is often quite independent of its efficacy. Thus, an instrument may perform its intended functions quite well while still being unsafe with regard to ground-current protection. Furthermore, the frequent needs to move instruments from one location to another and the possible variety of lead connections to patients may well create conditions under which hazards are not readily detected. Fortunately, the pertinent factors can be identified and equipments so designed that these hazards are minimized.

There are three ways for ground currents to enter or leave an instrument (Fig. 4-7), via the U-ground, the chassis ground, and the patient leads. The U-ground from the 3-prong 110-V plug is usually connected internally to the instrument chassis, and it carries stray currents from the instrument to the locale ground. Some instruments have a separate external grounding point, which is tied to the patient reference grounding bus. It can be a second potential path for stray ground currents. The remaining paths are via the patient leads, which can conduct currents either into or out of the instrument. Currents emanating from the instruments are generated by internal circuits or are a result of power-line leakage within the instrument. But hazard currents need not originate within the instrument. Currents could enter the instrument from the outside because the impedance of the patient leads to ground is unfavorably small.

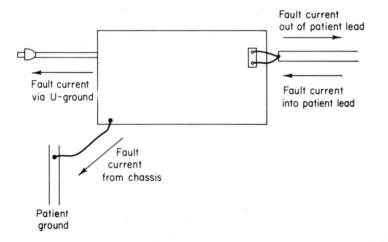

Fig. 4-7 Fault currents in instruments. Four common paths are via the U-ground in the power cord, via the chassis to an external ground, and in and out of patient leads.

Leakage currents from the input ac power lines are by far the most common cause for ground currents; these can be avoided by using battery-powered instruments, which accounts for their increasing popularity, particularly when such instruments are employed in connection with implanted devices. In line-powered instruments, the power transformer plays a crucial role in determining leakage currents.

A typical power transformer consists of an iron core on which several windings are mounted. Each winding is made of many turns of insulated copper wire and is totally insulated from the iron core and from the other windings. The power line is connected to one of these windings, the primary, and energy is transferred to the others by induction—not by direct metallic contact. Since the remaining windings are totally insulated from the primary, no direct path from the power lines to ground can (ideally) exist by way of these windings. Thus, power-line leakage currents occur principally from the primary windings and leads to ground and seldom occur elsewhere in the instrument. Transformers, however, are not ideal devices and, in addition to the inductive transfer of power, have some capacitances among the windings and to the core. Even though small, some ac current can flow through these capacitances.

Since the transformer is usually mounted on the chassis, this leakage current will find its way into the instrument ground. Fortunately, the transformer capacitance and therefore the leakage current can be controlled to a large degree by special precautions taken in the design of the transformer. A thin copper sheet may be placed around each winding and insulating material inserted between the copper sheets and the iron core. Electrostatic shields are thus created which reduce the capacitances among the windings and core and thus reduce leakage currents. These shields do not prevent the normal power transfer among the windings by induction.

The way in which the shields are connected affects the ground-current flow significantly. Consider Fig. 4-8, which shows several methods of connecting transformers to grounds. An instrument using a transformer without shield is shown in Fig. 4-8a. It is typical of older devices. For simplicity, only the connections to the primary winding of the transformer and the ground path from its iron core are shown. The transformer is mounted on the instrument chassis, which is also connected by wire to the U-ground of the input power plug. Thus, a path exists from the power line via the transformer capacitance to the iron core and back into the ground system of the locale. At times, one of the patient leads may also be connected to the instrument chassis. Under this condition, the path also leads through the patient to the locale ground. Also, the instrument chassis may be touched from the outside by some person, which creates still another path for ground currents.

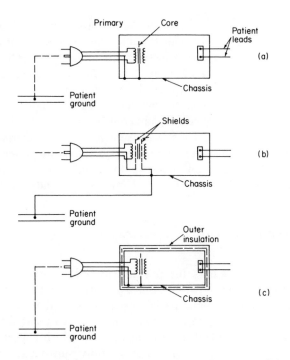

Fig. 4-8 Instrument grounding. (a) Conventional single-ground instrument. (b) Double-ground system. (c) Double-insulated equipment.

When an electrostatic shield is incorporated, as in Fig. 4-8b, there will be less leakage current among windings because the shield has reduced the interwinding capacitance. When the primary-winding shield is tied to the U-ground of the plug while the instrument chassis is not, the power-line leakage currents are effectively diverted away from the instrument chassis into the U-ground. The instrument chassis may then be grounded to the patient reference grounding bus, but only a minute fraction of the power line leakage will take this path. Even a patient lead tied to the instrument chassis will then carry very little leakage current.

Another alternative—using double insulation—is shown in Fig. 4-8c. The instrument chassis in this arrangement is totally protected from any contact with the outside, either directly or via patient leads, by an insulated case having a small enough capacitance to be safe. Very little of the leakage current present in the instrument chassis can then reach the patient or appear on the outside surface of the instrument, and much of the transformer shielding may therefore be avoided. The inner instrument chassis is still connected to the U-ground of the power plug, through which leakage currents are diverted.

Although the power transformer is the major source of leakage currents, it is by no means the only one. Because the sources of current leakage differ among the many types of instruments in use, specific details cannot be readily presented. Much of the protection in this connection is afforded by having all patient leads electrically isolated from the chassis and by establishing impedance levels to the chassis high enough so that leakage currents cannot inherently rise to dangerous values.

To reiterate, the fact that many instruments are moved from one place to another and are connected in different ways can create potentially hazardous situations that are not found in fixed installations. Especially for this reason, the need for frequent testing for good grounds is often stressed.

Interconnected Patient Systems

The NFPA requirements for patients in ESPA's stress an individual grounding system for each patient. Since no patient may be served by more than one grounding system, special precautions need to be taken when electrical connections to a locale outside of the patient's area are made. A good example is the central monitoring facility, which collects vital data from many patients. If grounding is not carefully controlled, stray currents can pass from one area to another by way of the monitoring equipment, and these currents could easily pass through one or more patients.

The intermixing of signals from different ground systems can be handled in various safe ways, some of which are shown in Fig. 4-9. In Fig. 4-9a, the patient output leads are ungrounded, each lead having a very high impedance to the local ground. The leads are connected to the balanced-input terminals of the monitoring device. This technique permits each device to be independently grounded to its own room. A second technique, shown in Fig. 4-9b, is used when the patient-monitoring instrument has a grounded output. In this case, only the signal lead is actually connected to the central monitor. The second, grounded lead of the output pair may be used as a shielded lead but must not be connected to any grounded point outside the patient area. The shielded lead serves to avoid picking up interference signals. Interfering signals may still appear on the monitor with this arrangement because a voltage difference may be present between the patient ground and the monitor ground, and this voltage will appear on the monitor superimposed upon the patient signal. This extraneous signal may well confuse the observer of the monitored output and could interfere with proper diagnosis. A third technique (Fig. 4-9c) avoids the disadvantage of grounded-output devices by inserting a photocoupler

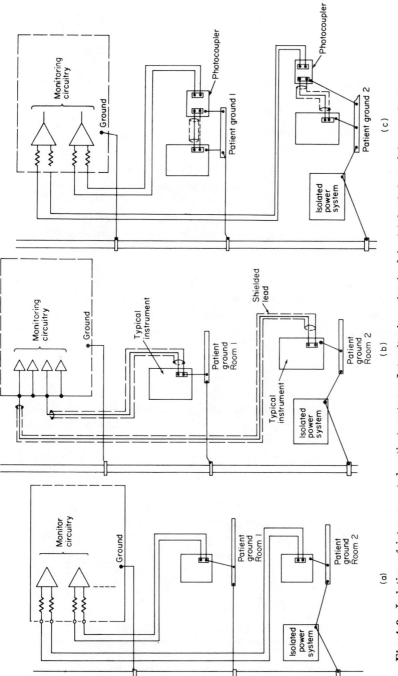

Fig. 4-9 Isolation of interconnected patient systems. Integrity is maintained in (a) by balanced inputs, in (b) by not connecting signal grounds at the monitor, and in (c) by using photocouplers.

between the patient-monitoring device and the central monitor. Such an isolator provides positive separation between the two ground systems because no metallic connection exists between input and output. Photo-coupling devices are discussed in Chapter 5 in the section dealing with semiconductor photosystems.

Power-Line Voltages

The many power-line receptacles in a building are not always supplied from the same secondary distribution system, and this may cause the voltage between nearby receptacles to rise above expected values. The possibilities are illustrated in Fig. 4-10, which shows a three-phase primary electric system supplying a large consumer such as a hospital. When the power is supplied from only one of the primary power lines, the recep-tacles will have voltages as shown on the three receptacles at the left. All the indicated measurements are between the ungrounded lines only. Each secondary distribution system is a 115/230-V cluster from which two distinct ungrounded lines emanate. All receptacles supplied from the same distribution lines are at the same potential and the voltage be-tween them is zero. But the voltages between the two ungrounded lines is 230 V.

The situation changes when more than one secondary distribution system is used, as may well be true in hospitals. For example, the power lines for the life-support branches may not come from the same primary winding as those in the life-safety branch, and the resultant interreceptacle voltages may be quite different from those just stated. The illustration shows three clusters of receptacles, each being energized by a different primary phase. The voltages appearing among the ungrounded lines of various receptacles are also shown, and these reveal a variety of possible voltages. Since leakage current is proportional to voltage, these variations may prove important in a given installation. It is obviously preferable to supply all power to a given patient from the same phase and preferably also from the same line in the secondary distribution system.

Standards and Specifications

The standards and specifications listed here are only those directly related to the text. For a more extensive listing, see A. F. Pacela, *A Guide to Biomedical Standards*, Second Edition, Quest Publishing Company, Diamond Bar, California, 1972.

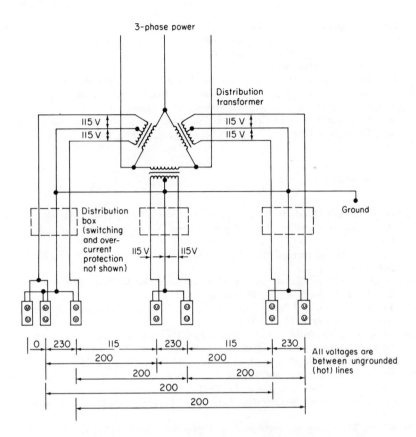

Fig. 4-10 Receptacle voltages in 115/230-V secondary distribution system. When receptacles are powered from more than one distribution box, voltages often exist between hot terminals of different receptacles. Voltages shown are for 3-phase primary power systems.

National Fire Protection Association, Boston, Massachusetts:

Publication 56A	Standard for the Use of Inhalation Anesthetics (Flammable and Nonflammable), 1971.
Publication 70	National Electrical Code, 1971.
Publication 76A	Standards for Essential Electrical Systems for Hospitals, 1971.
Publication 76BM	Manual for the Safe Use of Electricity in Hospitals, 1971.
Publication 76CM	Manual for the Safe Use of High-Frequency Electrical Equipment in Hospitals, 1970.

Pacela, A. F., Kemmer, A. F., and Lowery, A. Recommended AAMI Safety Standard for Electromedical Apparatus—Part 1, Safe Current Limits, *J. AAMI*, **4**, 132, 1970; revised Feb. 1971.

Underwiters Laboratories, Inc., Melville, New York:
  Subject 544   Medical and Dental Equipment Intended for Use in Non-Hazardous
    Areas, Fourth Draft, 1971.
Veterans Administration, Washington, D.C.:
  Biomedical Monitoring Systems: Electro-Biometrics for Intensive-Care Units, VA
    Specification X-1414, Jan. 1, 1970, Amendment No. 1, Sept. 1, 1970.
Department of Health, Education, and Welfare, Washington, D.C.:
  General Standards of Construction and Equipment for Hospital and Medical Facili-
    ties, Public Health Service Publ., No. 930-A-7, revised Feb. 1969.

Bibliography

Arnow, S., Bruner, J. M. R., Siegal, E. F., and Sloss, L. J., Ventricular Fibrillation
  Associated with an Electrically Operated Bed, *New England J. Med.* **281**, No. 1
  (July 1969).
Battig, C. G., Electrosurgical Burn Injuries and their Prevention, *J. Amer. Med. Ass.*
  204 (June 1968).
Bekink, J., The Prevention of Leakage Currents in Special Medical Care Rooms, *Elec-
  trotechniek* (Neth., in Dutch) **49**, No. 25 (1971).
Ben-Zvi, S., The Lack of Safety Standards in Medical Instrumentation, *Trans. N.Y.
  Acad. Sci. Ser. II* **31** (June 1969).
Bibliography on Electrical Hazards, Safety and Standards in Biomedical Engineering,
  Beckman Instruments Inc., Fullerton, California Rep. CCR-21A (July 1970).
Billin, A. G., Patient Safety and Electrosurgery, *AORN J.* (Aug. 1971).
Bousvaros, G. A., Don, C., and Hopps, J. A., An Electric Hazard of Selective Angio-
  cardiography, *Can. Med. Ass. J.* **87** (1962).
Bruner, J. M., Hazards of Electrical Apparatus, *Anesthesiology* **28**, No. 2 (Mar./Apr.
  1967).
Bucher, P., The Safety of Electromedical Equipment, *Elektroniker* (Germany, in Ger-
  man) **10**, No. 1 (Feb. 1971).
Burchell, H. B., Hidden Hazards of Cardiac Pacemakers, *Circulation* **24** (1961).
Burchell, H. B., Electrocution Hazards in the Hospital or Laboratory, *Circulation* **27**
  (1963).
Burchell, H. B., and Sturm, R. E., Electroshock Hazards, *Circulation* **35** (1967).
Burns from Needle Electrodes of Electrocardiogram Monitor, (Clinical Anesth. Conf.)
  N.Y. State J. Med. **68** (1968).
Cartwright, J., and Widginton, D. W., Safety Barriers for use in Intrinsically Safe
  Circuits, *Conf. Elect. Safety Hazard. Environment, London* (1971).
Cheorghiu, P., Electric Hazards and Safety in Medical Instrumentation, *Proc. Annu.
  Conf. Eng. Med. Biol. IEEE Houston* **10** (1968).
Claxton, R. E., Remember Standby Power, *Allis-Chalmer Eng. Rev.* **34**, No. 2 (1969).
Danger of Sparking and the Measurement of the Inherent Safety When Using Electro-
  medical Equipment which Employs Electrode and Intercardial Catheters, *Alta
  Freq. Suppl.* (Italy, in Italian), **75**, No. 5 (May 1971).
Dangers in Poorly Designed Medical Electronic Equipment (Editorial), *N.Y. State J.
  Med.* **68**, 1915 (1968).
Deb, A. K., Electrical Shock Hazards and Safety of Patients and Operators in Intensive
  Care Units, *Electrotechnology (India)* **14**, No. 2 (Mar./Apr. 1970).

Dobbie, A. K., Electricity in Hospitals, *Biomed. Eng (GB)* **7**, No. 1 (1972).

Dolling, H. F. H., Application of the Total-Energy Concept to Hospital Electricity Generation and Steam Boiler Plants, *Hosp. Eng. (GB)* **24** (Dec. 1970).

Doyle, O., Designers of Medical Instruments Face Serious Questions on Safety, *Electronics* **42**, 4 (1969).

Electric Hazards in Hospitals, Nat. Acad. Sci. (1970).

Emergency Generating Sets, *Tech. Mod.* (France, in French) **62**, No. 1 (Jan. 1970).

Eriqat, A. K., Four Power Sources Insure Hospital Safety, *Electron. Constr. Maint.* **69**, No. 12 (Dec. 1970).

French, H., Medical Electronic Equipment and Hospital Safety, *Pop. Electron. Incl. Electron World* **1**, No. 1 (1972).

Gibbs, D. B., Medical Electronic Systems Demand Careful Planning, *Can. Electron. Eng.* **16**, No. 4 (Apr. 1972).

Graystone, P., Electrical Safety in Hospitals, *Can. Hosp. 5th Annu. Constr. Planning Issue, 5th* (1973).

Griffin, N. L., Electronics for Hospital Patient Care, U.S. Dept. HEW, Publ. Health Serv. Publ. No. 930-D-25. U.S. Govt. Printing Office, Washington, D.C.

Holm, R., "Electrical Contacts Handbook." Springer-Verlag, Berlin and New York, 1958.

Hopps, J. A., Electrical Hazards in Hospitals, *Bull. Radio EE Div., NRC* **20**, No. 2 (Apr. 1970).

Jedynak, L., Where the (Switch) Action Is, *IEEE Spectrum* **10**, No. 10 (Oct. 1973).

Jones, F. L., "The Physics of Electrical Contacts." Oxford Univ. Press (Clarendon), London and New York, 1957.

Kaufmann, R. H., Important Functions Performed by an Effective Equipment Grounding System, *IEEE Trans. Ind. Gen. Appl.* **IGA-6**, No. 6 (Nov./Dec. 1970).

Klomp, A. M., and Lucas, J. H. M., Considerations on the Safety of Electrical Equipment in Medical Practice for the Preparation of an International Standard, Eurocon 71 Digest, IEEE, Lausanne, Switzerland (1971).

Leonard, P. F., and Gould, A. B., Dynamics of Electrical Hazards of Particular Concern to Operating-Room Personnel, *Surg. Clin. N. Amer.* **45**, 817 (1965).

Link, D. M., Current Regulatory Aspects of Medical Devices, *IEEE Proc. 1972 Annu. Reliabil. Maint. Symp., San Francisco* (1972).

Medical Electronics and Data, Safety Issue (Nov./Dec. 1970).

Medicine and the Law: Fatal Shock from a Cardiac Monitor, *Lancet* **1**, 872 (1960).

Meyer, J. A., Electrical Hazards in Medical Instrumentation, *Clin. Anesth.* **5**, 53 (1967).

Miller, W. B., Safety of Electrical Systems in Operating Rooms, *Cn. Hosp.* **44** (1967).

Mody, S. M., and Richings, M., Ventricular Fibrillation Resulting from Electrocution during Cardiac Catheterization, *Lancet* **2** (Oct. 6, 1962).

NASA, Aerospace Technology and Hospital Systems, NASA Technology Utilization Office, Southwest Res. Inst., San Antonio, Texas.

Pacela, A. F., Design of Medical Electronic Equipment for Patient Safety, *IEEE WESCON Tech Papers* **14** (1970).

Pocock, S. N., Earth-Free Patient Monitoring, *Biomed. Eng* **7**, No. 1 (1972).

Soares, E. C., "Grounding Electrical Distribution Systems for Safety." Marsh Publ., Wayne, New Jersey (1968).

Spencer, E. W., Ingram, V. M., and Levinthal, C., Electrophoresis: An Accident and Some Precautions, *Science* **152**, 1722 (1966).

Standby Diesel Electricity Generating Plant, *Hosp. Eng. (GB)* **24** (Sept. 1970).

Stanley, P. E., Monitors That Save Lives Can Also Kill, *Mod. Hosp.* **108** (Mar. 1967).

Stanley, P. E., Hospital Electrical Safety and Shielding, *J. Ass. Advan. Med. Instrum* **2** (Mar./Apr. 1967).

Vickers, M. D., Explosion Hazards in Anaesthesia, *Anaesthesia* **25**, No. 4 (Oct. 1970).

Wakely, W. N., Some Aspects of Medical Electronics, *Hosp. Eng.* (*GB*) **24**, No. 8 (Aug. 1970).

Wald, A., Mazzia, V. D. B., and Spencer, F. C., Accidental Burns Associated with Electrocautery, *J. Amer. Med. Ass.* (Aug. 1971).

Walter, C. W., Anesthetic Explosions: a Continuing Threat, *Anesthesiology* **25**, 505 (1964).

Walter, C. W., Fire in an Oxygen-Powered Respirator, *J. Amer. Med. Ass.* **197**, No. 1 (1966).

Watson, A. C., Emergency Power Systems for Hospitals, *Hosp. Eng.* (*GB*) **23**, No. 6 (June 1969).

Weinberg, D. I., Electrical Safety in the Operating Room and at the Bedside, "Engineering in the Practice of Medicine." Williams and Wilkins, Baltimore, Maryland, 1967.

Whalen, R. E., Starmer, C. F., and McIntosh, H. D., Electrical Hazards Associated with Cardiac Pacemakers, *Ann. N.Y. Acad. Sci.* **111** (1964).

Whalen, R. E., Starmer, C. F., and McIntosh, H. D., Electric Shock Hazards in Clinical Cardiology, *Mod. Conc. Cardiovasc. Dis.* **36** (1967).

Wilke, H., Considerations on an Emergency Power Generation Unit, *Energ. U. Tech.* (Germany, in German) **21**, No. 1 (Sept. 1969).

Chapter 5

PATIENT-PROTECTION SYSTEMS

This chapter is devoted to the description of several devices designed specifically to provide safety protection for patients.

Patient-Lead Devices

The earlier discussions have dealt largely with grounding and the means to ensure a safe patient environment by good grounding. The patient, however, is connected to patient leads. These leads normally carry diagnostic or therapeutic signals from or to the patient, and they could be contaminated with accidental signals or voltages other than those intended. Safety hazards might thereby arise.

An alteration of the normal patient signal may be due to many causes. First, there may be possible signal changes due to the existence of voltage drops among grounds; protection against this hazard has already been described. Second, a change may occur in the level or the nature of the normal signal delivered from instrument to patient. Well-designed instruments provide signals, however, that do not change substantially over long periods of use. Other causes might be the development of faults within an instrument. If, for example, a portion of the power-line current were to appear on the patient lead, excessive patient-lead current could well result. The current flow does not have to be due to the instrument from which the patient lead emanates, as shown in Fig. 5-1, but could also result from another instrument in which a fault has occurred. The patient lead might then conduct fault currents into ground. This condition can be alleviated by having adequately large impedance levels within the instrument to ground, or by the use of patient-lead devices.

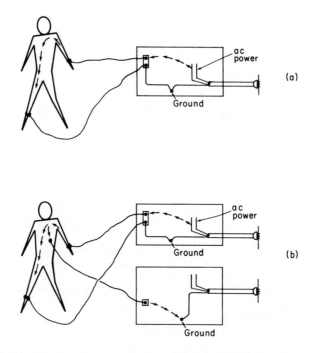

Fig. 5-1 Causes for excessive patient-lead current. A fault or leakage from power lines to the patient terminal might occur, (a) sending current through the patient; or an instrument might conduct dangerous currents from patient to ground (b).

The patient-lead devices discussed here are intended to provide protection against the flow of excessive patient-lead current in either direction from any source. Three techniques will be discussed—current limiters, signal isolation devices, and fuses.

Current limiters use electronic components to limit the maximum amount of current in the patient lead to a predetermined, safe value. The maximum current is determined by the physical properties of semiconductors and, as long as these devices are protected from failure and burnout, good protection is afforded.

Signal-isolation devices use circuit-coupling methods that isolate the instrument terminals completely from the patient leads so that no metallic connection exists between them. When a fault develops on the instrument side of the device, excessive currents that might then be present in the signal leads will not be transferred across the isolation system. Patient-lead currents can thus be held within safe limits.

Fuses in patient leads are designed to burn out upon prolonged application of currents in excess of the fuse rating. Only then is the path via the patient lead disrupted. This delay represents the principal shortcoming of fuses as patient-protection devices.

A. Current Limiters

One method of current limiting involves semiconductor diodes. A diode conducts current in only one direction. During this forward conduction, the voltage drop across the diode is nearly constant. At a very small magnitude of forward current, however, as current is increased from zero, the voltage does increase, until it reaches its constant forward voltage drop. In the reverse direction, no conduction takes place until the voltage exceeds the specified rating of the diode, after which heavy conduction commences. These characteristics are shown in the voltage curves of Fig. 5-2a. When two diodes are reverse-connected as in Fig. 5-2b, the combined curves act to limit voltages of both positive and negative polarity. Reverse-connected diodes are therefore used whenever fault currents might be either positive or negative, or ac. The forward drop of a semiconductor diode is determined by the materials of which the diode is made and is fixed for a given material. The most commonly used silicon devices have a drop of 0.7 V per diode. For germanium, a less suitable material, this drop is 0.2 V. This limitation also restricts the normal patient signals to under 0.7 V for silicon unless several diodes are connected in series, which arrangement multiplies the limiting voltage levels. An example of this approach is shown in Fig. 5-2c. Unless a great number of additional diodes are used, the permitted voltage levels on patient leads cannot be more than a few volts. Thus, the usefulness of this type of protection device is limited to only those instruments in which small signal levels are conveyed.

In practical applications of diodes as limiters, the diodes cannot simply be connected across the patient leads without further circuitry, for under abnormal conditions a fault current might develop that could cause the diode current ratings to be exceeded. Diodes must be protected from this possibility, or burnout with its consequent loss of protection will result. The addition of resistors in patient leads serves this need. Whereas the diodes do not interfere with the normal transmission of patient signals, the added resistors reduce signal magnitude. Such a loss in signal level is a serious disadvantage whenever signals are inherently tiny in magnitude, as in EKG equipment. Figure 5-3 shows three current-limiter arrangements of the resistance–diode type.

Another type of current limiter results in reduced resistances and therefore less loss of signal. This scheme uses field-effect diodes and tran-

sistors (connected as diodes), which are also known as constant-current
diodes, current zeners, and regulator diodes. As the voltage is increased
across these devices, current at first also increases. At some voltage, the
current levels off to an essentially constant value which is maintained as the
voltage is further increased. A typical current–voltage curve for two
such devices connected back to back is given in Fig. 5-4a. The important
quantity is the limiting current, which is predetermined by selection of the
semiconductor device and which must be chosen small enough to constitute
a safe level of patient current. Such devices may be connected is series,
which multiplies the allowable signal voltage, or in parallel, for additional

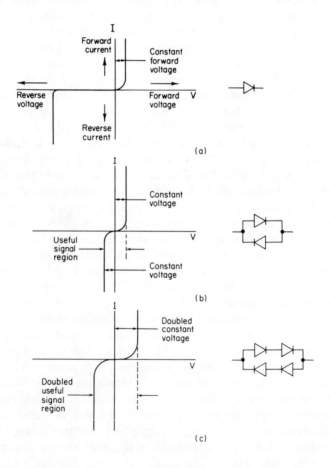

Fig. 5-2 Diodes as protective devices. (a) Typical current–voltage curve. (b)
Voltage limiting with reverse-connected diodes. (c) Doubling the voltage where limiting
occurs by doubling the number of diodes.

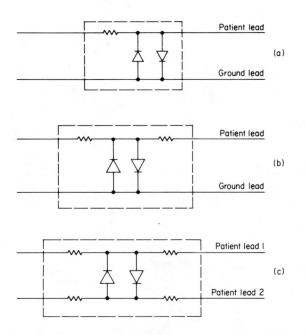

Fig. 5-3 Resistance–diode current limiter. Arrangement (a) protects only against faults originating from the left side, (b) protects from both directions. Both (a) and (b) are for single-ended, grounded patient leads, (c) is for balanced, ungrounded patient leads.

current-carrying ability. For the latter, the limiting current value of the combination must be held within safe limits. As with the earlier configuration, protection must be added against component burnout, in this case by use of resistors and zener diodes. A complete patient-lead circuit using field-effect diodes is shown in Fig. 5-4b. Additional details and examples of both circuit types described in this section are given in Appendix G.

B. *Signal-Isolation Devices*

Although current limiters are able to protect patients and instruments from accidental hazards on signal leads, their protection does not extend to faulty interconnection of grounding systems; such hazards may still exist, therefore, even though current limiters are used. In order to make further improvements in isolating grounds from patients and instruments, techniques for transmitting electrical information by means other than a metallic connection are being increasingly explored. There are two general

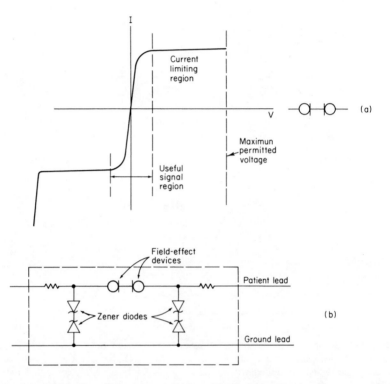

Fig. 5-4 Field-effect-diode current limiter. (a) Typical current–voltage curve for a back-to-back connected field-effect-diode pair. (b) Complete protection arrangement for single-ended, grounded patient leads.

methods for transmitting electrical data without metallic interconnection—coupling magnetically or by electromagnetic radiation. Figure 5-5 shows the two basic schemes.

Magnetic coupling requires a transformer or coil, but the frequency characteristics of the signal in many applications are not fully compatible with those required by the magnetic device. Hence, the incoming signal must first be made compatible with the characteristics of the magnetic device. This task is performed by a signal conditioner such as a modulator. After the signal energy has been transferred via the magnetic device, it must, in many cases, again be restored to its original condition by means of a restorer such as a demodulator. The difficulties and therefore the expense associated with the use of magnetic coupling are usually due to the complexities of these auxiliary devices. For example, to transfer information having a bandwidth of up to 50 kHz may well require a complicated modulating system in which the entire information to be transferred is first modulated upon a high-frequency carrier, then transferred by means of a radio-frequency coil, and finally demodulated. Not only is this process costly but, because of its power consumption, it makes more difficult the use of batteries for energization. Batteries, it may be recalled, are necessary if interconnection of the input and output grounding systems is to be avoided, because common power systems introduce common grounds and thereby negate the effectiveness of the scheme.

The second method for transferring electrical energy without metallic interconnection involves radiated energy. Coupling may be achieved by radio-frequency energy, like radio transmission into our homes, or by other forms of electromagnetic radiation. The most common energy transfer in instrumentation takes place by means of a light beam, the intensity of which is varied in accordance with the signal being transferred. Each such coupling unit utilizes a light source the output of which is observed by a nearby photodetector. Examples of light sources are incandescent bulbs, photolamps, and infrared emitters. Among detectors are the solar cells and phototransistors. In general, the problems of conditioning and restoring the signal information are quite similar to those of the magnetic coupling systems, but an additional problem is the heat generated by the light source, which can reflect itself not only in local heating and consequently reduced instrument reliability but also in excess power consumption, which affects battery life.

Until recently, few nonmetallic transfer systems were in use because their disadvantages often outweighed their potential improvements, especially with regard to excessive bulk, power consumption, and cost. Recently, a number of devices have been developed that remove many of the objections to earlier practical systems. These devices—semiconductor light-emitting diodes coupled to phototransistors—actually come close to

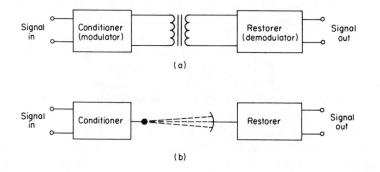

Fig. 5-5 Nonmetallic transfer of signals. (a) Magnetic coupling. (b) Radiated energy.

achieving the objectives of good signal compatibility, excellent isolation, reliable life, small size and power consumption, and low cost. It is expected that these devices will find increasing use in biomedical instrumentation, since they promise to achieve a degree of potential patient safety not heretofore practically possible.

Semiconductor Photosystems   The basic elements of the semiconductor light source is a light-emitting diode that, upon the application of very small currents (a few milliamperes), emits infrared light of sufficient strength that it may be detected by a sensor positioned a fraction of an inch away from the light source. The radiating wavelength depends upon the semiconductor materials chosen: currently available gallium arsenide diodes emit near 0.9 μm, gallium arsenide phosphide near 0.65 μm, and gallium phosphide near 0.7 μm. The detector is also a semiconductor device, usually of silicon, either a diode or a transistor, the current flow within which varies with optical excitation. The wavelength bands over which the detectors are sensitive are wider than those of the light sources and usually cover the emission band of light-emitting diodes.

Both types of device are commercially marketed separately and may be individually applied at the designer's choice. One of the more useful devices, however, combines the light-emitting diode with a phototransistor in an integral package, the device being known as a photodetector coupler, or an optical coupler. Figure 5-6a shows typical characteristics of this device. For biomedical applications relating to safety, the isolation of the input from the output is most significant, some units now available having isolation to 5000 V. To ensure patient safety, the insulation resistance must also be controlled so that it is never less than the ratio of the maximum anticipated fault voltage (a pulsed defibrillator, for example) to the safe patient current. This requirement usually dictates that the insulation resistance be at least 10^9 ohms. For the same reason, capacitance across the optical interface must also be small to avoid significant energy transfer.

The great advantages of the optical coupler are (1) its small power dissipation and (2) its compatibility with instrumentation signals, which obviates the need for extensive signal conditioning and restoration. As may be seen from Figs. 5-6b and 5-6c, the device may be directly coupled to the integrated-circuit logic gates and drivers, for purely digital data transfer, and to operational amplifiers for linear circuit applications. (The detailed circuit components for the operational amplifiers have been omitted in Fig. 5-6c.) Contrasted to other light sources, the photocoupling system is also much superior with regard to lamp life. The transfer limitations of the photocoupling device lie in the areas of signal bandwidth, slew rate, rise and fall times, and delays. At the present time, bandwidths

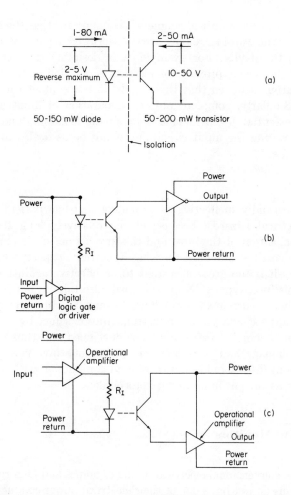

Fig. 5-6 Photocoupler energy transfer. (a) Typical device characteristics. Bandwidth to 2 MHz; slew rate as small as 0.15 V/μsec; rise time, fall time, and delays several microseconds. Vertical dashed line: isolation to 5000 V; insulation resistance 10^{10} to 10^{13} ohms. (b) Digital circuit configuration. (c) Linear circuit configuration.

up to several megahertz have been achieved, which permit the coupler to be used in EKG, EEG, and many other applications without impairing signal quality. In some applications, where signal amplitudes change over relatively large ranges, the slew rate may become a limiting factor, slowing down the responses to large signal changes. However, because of the relatively small bandwidth requirements of EKG and EEG signals, slew rate is not important in these applications.

In the application of optical couplers it is important that the advantages accruing from the use of the device are not sacrificed in part by the methods of applying the device. For example, it is desirable that the packages selected for the device provide for physical separation of the input leads from the output leads so that these leads do not contact each other accidentally. Similarly, complete physical separation of input and output circuits is essential for achieving safe circuit isolation, and of course batteries powering the input circuits must not be used also to power the output circuits.

C. *Fuses*

Fuses are usually ineffective in providing first-line patient protection against electrical hazards, because of the relatively long time elapsed between application of the fault and the fuse action in disconnecting the circuit. The smallest standard fuse has a current capacity of $\frac{1}{500}$ amp, which by itself is too great a current to be effective against microshock hazards. This fuse, type AGX or AGC, will also take as much as 5 sec to burn out when a current of 4 mA flows through the fuse. However, fuses play important secondary roles in instrumentation safety by disconnecting critical circuits shortly after a fault has developed and thus can prevent equipment damage and fires. For all applications involving patient instrumentation, fuses should be used only in conjunction with other safety devices such as current limiters or photocouplers.

Ground Monitors

Unlike the conventional electrical wiring of homes and factories, isolated power systems do not have one of their electrical power conductors tied to ground. The reasons for this have been described earlier. When a fault develops from one power line to ground, the electric circuit from one power line to the other is not completed because neither power line is grounded. This has the advantage that a spark, which the same fault might cause in a grounded system, cannot develop. A second fault or a leakage path from the other power line, however, will complete the circuit path, and such a combination of faults could cause sparking to take place. In order to preclude this condition, it is essential that the occurrence of the first be detected. Fortunately, this can be done by means of ground monitors.

Ground monitors sense the changes occurring in ground currents that result from the development of faults from power lines to ground. The monitors are generally able to discriminate between normally expected leakage currents and fault currents, and they provide the necessary warnings early enough to forestall more serious problems later. The protection afforded by these devices is often stated in terms of fault impedance. Whenever the impedance from power line to ground becomes less than the rated, predetermined fault impedance, the current flow via the fault is judged to be excessive and the alarm is activated.

Ground monitors have been required for many years in hospital facilities where flammable anesthetics are used and where the risk of a spark in connection with electrical faults could easily present a serious explosion hazard. By monitoring the ground current, they seek to measure the degree of isolation actually present in the isolated power lines. The fault current from power line to ground (or from one power line to the other) is not the same as the ground current being monitored, and the two currents are not even necessarily proportional to each other. Their relationship depends upon the type of monitor selected.

The ground monitor is expected to signal the occurrence of all important abnormal conditions within the isolated power system. In flammable-anesthetics locations, these must necessarily include all faults due to which sparking might occur. Recently, isolated power systems have also been considered as protective devices against microshock. The monitor needs then to detect every occurrence of excessive ground-current flow. This criterion is quite different from that applicable to flammable anesthetics, and different types of ground monitors, such as passive detectors, may detect excessive ground currents more readily. No suitable ground monitors for protection against microshock are presently available because existing devices by themselves cause a large enough ground current to constitute a microshock hazard. The succeeding discussions therefore address themselves primarily to systems used where flammable anesthetics may be present.

A ground monitor consists of a measuring device that is coupled to the ungrounded power leads of an isolated power system in order to measure in some manner all the current flow to ground. It does not actually measure fault currents from the power lines— only ground currents resulting therefrom. However, when ground current increases to a level above that normally anticipated, a power-line fault is presumed to have occurred. Most ground monitors are so arranged that no ground current flows under normal conditions. As soon as stray currents exist or some fault develops within the monitor's sensing capability, some current will flow through the detector portion of the monitor. The fault current causing this ground current may or may not constitute a hazard, depending upon its magnitude. An alarm system is normally associated with the ground monitor, which is activated whenever the detector current exceeds a predetermined threshold value. This alarm may activate an audible tone, a signal light, or both, or it may be used to disconnect the electric power to the facility.

Two basic schemes for detecting line faults are shown in Fig. 5-7. One of these, in Fig. 5-7a, depends upon the assumption that unless all current flowing in one power line returns by way of the other, a leakage path must be present that shunts off a portion of the current via a third path, presumably ground. Thus, it monitors each of the power lines out of the isolation transformers, perhaps by means of a magnetic coupling loop, and performs a subtraction of the two currents. In the absence of trouble, the difference should be zero.

The second scheme, in Fig. 5-7b, establishes an electric voltage point midway between that of the two power lines, and monitors the voltage from this point to ground. Since it is prearranged that this voltage point is approximately at ground potential, very little or no detector current normally flows. It is thus possible to detect unbalanced conditions resulting

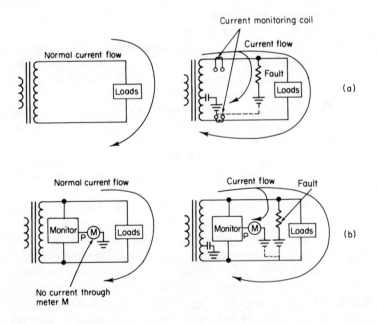

Fig. 5-7 Two methods of line-isolation monitoring. (a) Current sensing: difference between current flow in the two power leads. (b) Voltage sensing: difference of potential between an artificial ground at P and the actual ground.

from leakage currents or faults. This second scheme, using voltage sensing, is extensively used in hospitals.

Each of the two methods has its own advantages and limitations. The first one senses current and thus permits magnetic coupling to be used. The entire sensing circuit is then electrically isolated from the remaining system, thereby protecting the patient from the possibility of hazard currents being introduced by the detection device. There are practical difficulties, however, in using this technique. They arise because the faults to be detected represent only a minute fraction of the total power-line currents. Depending on the size of the isolated power system, normal currents range from 5 to 30 amp, while the fault currents to be detected are as small as 1 mA. This ratio, up to 30,000:1, taxes the component tolerances, necessitating critical adjustments, and tends to make the device sensitive to stray interfering currents due to sudden load changes and due to stray capacitive leakage currents from the isolation transformer. This method is also insensitive to those faults during which fault currents return only by way of the power lines, although the latter do not generally constitute a hazard to the patient.

Voltage sensing, on the other hand, has the advantage of being able to detect all types of faults but suffers from its direct interconnection into the power and ground system. The direct connection permits the detector circuitry to contribute an additional small current into the ground system, which obviously tends to increase any already existing hazard.

A. Voltage-Sensing Systems

The prevalent circuit in voltage-sensing ground monitors is a version of the familiar Wheatstone bridge, shown in Fig. 5-8. This circuit has two branches; one consists of resistances R_1 and R_2 which are joined at point a, while the other uses resistances R_3 and R_4, joined at point b. In the absence of a connection between a and b, the input voltage E causes current I_a to flow in one branch, the magnitude of which is determined entirely by the sum of the two resistances in the branch. The second current I_b in the other branch is similarly determined by its two resistances. According to Ohm's law, each current causes a voltage drop to develop across each resistance. Thus, current I_a develops voltage $I_a R_2$ from a to c, and current I_b develops voltage $I_b R_4$ from b to c; and with some combinations of resistances these two voltages may be equal. When the voltages are equal, points a and b are at the same potential, and any electrical circuit then connected from a to b will be inactive. Thus, when a resistance R_5 is interposed from a to b, there will, in fact, be no current flow, and a metering device placed from a to b will register no current flow. This condition is

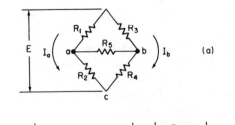

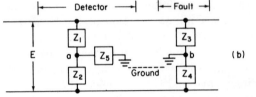

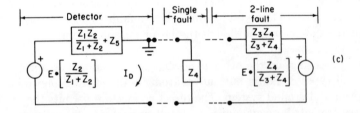

Fig. 5-8 Basic bridge circuit. (a) Wheatstone bridge. (b) Analogous line-isolation monitor circuit. (c) Equivalent circuit (see Chapter 2).

the balanced state of the Wheatstone bridge. In general, however, the five resistances need not be such that a balance is obtained, and there will then occur a current flow through resistance R_5 which depends upon the voltage from a to b. For ac circuits, the arms of the bridge are impedances made of combinations of resistances, inductances, and capacitances.

The ground monitor acts as a portion of such a Wheatstone bridge circuit, as shown in Fig. 5-8b, with impedances Z_1, Z_2, and Z_5 constituting the major elements of the system. As shown in the diagram, the system ground becomes a portion of the central leg of the bridge circuit, and ground current is sensed by means of a current-measuring device placed in the ground lead, represented by impedance Z_5. The bridge circuit is completed if faults occur, as represented by impedances Z_3 and Z_4. Probable faults may take many forms, resulting at times in various mixes of the values of Z_3 and Z_4, or the presence of only one or the other of the two. The circuit could then look like a Wheatstone bridge with one side removed, and balance under this condition is impossible.

A ground monitor may experience fault conditions for which Z_3 and Z_4 are such that the bridge is balanced. No alarm is then activated, even though a true fault may be present. This undesirable condition in ground monitors is termed the *blind spot*.

B. *Static and Dynamic Detectors*

The possibility that a line fault may be present but remain undetected by the ground monitor is intrinsic to the device so far depicted. The configuration is termed a *static detector*. Without altering the circuit substantially, another configuration, termed the *dynamic detector*, may be employed; it acts in a similar manner but does not have a blind spot. Both circuits are shown for comparison in Fig. 5-9. The dynamic detector uses a switching technique by which the detector is connected, alternately, to one or another set of impedances so that the detector current consists of two separately determined current components. As seen in Fig. 5-9b, switch S is connected first to point P for some period of time, and is then switched to point Q for a similar period. The switching process is then repeated regularly, with one or the other connection being made at all times. By proper choice of the impedances, at least one bridge will always be unbalanced and no blind spot will exist.

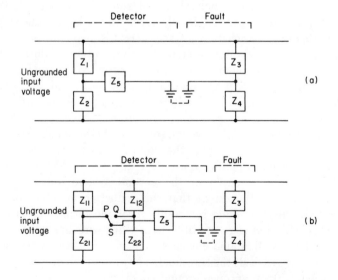

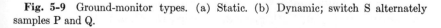

Fig. 5-9 Ground-monitor types. (a) Static. (b) Dynamic; switch S alternately samples P and Q.

C. *Passive and Active Detectors*

It is possible to insert a separate power source into the central leg of the bridge circuit and thereby alter the behavior of the ground monitor. Because the detector circuitry then contains a source of power, the detector is termed an *active detector*. There is no restriction placed upon what kind of power source this might be. Thus, in addition to power sources at power-line frequencies, power at totally different frequencies may prove to be useful. Although there is considerable potential to this type of detector, it is not presently widely used. Circuits not having the additional power source are called *passive detectors*.

For a more detailed treatment of voltage-sensing ground monitors, refer to Appendix H.

Ground-Continuity Monitors

Loss of ground represents probably the most serious cause of patient hazards, and it is not surprising that attention has recently been directed to ways of automatically monitoring grounds and detecting breaks in ground paths before they can cause damage. The efforts have been hampered by the need to provide this monitoring in a manner that will not itself add to the potential hazards of instrument installations. Practical systems can be either passive, in which no energy is introduced into the ground path, or active, whereby a trace current is used to assess continuity.

There are several ways of accomplishing ground-fault continuity monitoring. One technique monitors the voltage drop over a small segment of the grounding conductor in the line cord, amplifies it, and causes an alarm to be activated when the sensed voltage exceeds a predetermined threshold. Since the dc resistance across which monitoring takes place determines how much voltage drop will develop, some small additional resistance may be introduced intentionally into the ground system. This resistance will positively overcome amplifier noise, but any such additional resistance decreases the safety margin of the ground system under unfavorable fault conditions. To the extent that this reduction in safety margin can be tolerated, this technique represents a simple means for ground-continuity checking, and is compatible with three-wire line cords. The amplifier also detects all ground currents from whatever source whenever the amplified voltage exceeds the threshold. The system can also be arranged to sound an alarm upon an open-ground condition.

Another technique makes use of a fourth conductor in the line cord for an additional ground. Both grounds are tied together at the instrument,

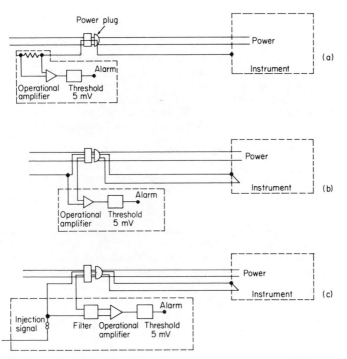

Fig. 5-10   Ground-continuity monitors. (a) Passive 3-wire version. (b) Passive 4-wire version. (c) Active 4-wire injection system.

and their voltage differences are monitored near the power plug. An open circuit or a large voltage difference will again cause an amplifier output to exceed its threshold and cause an alarm to be activated. The need for the fourth conductor makes this arrangement less practical than the one described earlier.

More positive indications can be obtained from a 4-wire system by injecting a current into one ground lead and monitoring this current in the other. The selection of a suitable frequency and amplitude which will not constitute a hazard to patients nor affect instrumentation adversely is difficult to accomplish. Figure 5-10 shows these configurations in more detail.

Bibliography

Bergey, G. E., and Squires, R. D. (UNADC), Improved Buffer Amplifier for Incorporation Within a Biopotential Electrode, *IEEE Trans. Biomed. Eng.* **BME-18,** No. 6 (Nov. 1971).

Bracale, M., Photon-Coupling in Biomedical Amplifiers, *Proc. Automat. Instrum. Conf.*, *11th, Milan* (1970).

Dalziel, J., Ground Fault Interrupter Increases Safety, *IAEI News* (July 1969).

Fish, R. M., The Use of Constant-Current Diodes in Preventing Electrical Shock from Hospital Equipment, *IEEE Trans. Biomed. Eng.* **BME-18,** No. 6 (Nov. 1971).

Gragstone, P., Ground Hazard Indicators, *Can. Hosp.* (Feb. 1973).

Holsinger, W. P., and Kempner, K. M. (NIH), Patient Electrode Isolation Adapter, *IEEE Trans. Biomed. Eng.* **BME-18,** No. 6 (Nov. 1971).

Huening, W. C., Jr., Aspects of Isolated Power Systems for Hospital Operating Rooms, *IEEE Trans. Ind. Gen. Appl.* (July 1965).

Kusters, N. L., The Ground Detector Problem in Hospital Operating Rooms, *Trans. EIC (Canada)* **2,** No. 1 (Jan. 1958).

McKinley, D. W. R., An Electronic Ground Detector, *Trans. EIC (Canada)* **2,** No. 1 (Jan. 1958).

Nestor, D. W., The Ground Fault Circuit Interrupter, *1970 I & CPS ESHAC Joint Tech. Conf.* (May 1970).

Otsuka, W. M., and Hunt, R. A., Sr., Innovations with Light Emitting Diodes, *IEEE WESCON Tech Papers* **14** (1970).

Walter, C. W., New Concept: Safe Patient Power Centre, *Modern Hospital* (June 1969).

Zicko, C. P., New Applications Open Up for the Versatile Isolation Amplifier, *Electronics* **45,** No. 7 (1972).

Chapter 6

SAFETY TESTING

Installation Testing

The principles and good practices underlying electrical safety have been described in the earlier chapters. This chapter addresses itself to the problem of how to ensure the continuous existence of safe conditions by testing. Safety testing in installations has two distinct phases: the initial test programs for new and modified installations, and the verification programs necessary to ensure continued safety.

The necessity for frequent testing arises from the continuously changing conditions in a normal health-care environment, where instruments and personnel are constantly moved and rearranged, and where a safe condition one day cannot be assumed to exist the next day. If all the equipments were rigidly mounted in one location, safety problems would be far less likely and an occasional safety check might well suffice. Some permanently installed fixtures and the electrical power-distribution systems are, of course, in this category, and they require relatively little attention. The bulk of the problem concerns the portable instruments, carried from room to room, plugged in and out of receptacles, handled at times with care but also occasionally mishandled. Since there are many such instruments, the desirable safety testing may be quite extensive in scope so that emphasis needs to be placed upon speedy testing. This is best done with test instruments capable of showing the test results in easily readable ways. Particularly useful is a category of test instruments which display the results either as GO or NO-GO, perhaps by means of lights; these instruments can readily be used by personnel otherwise untrained in electrical technology. This may permit some of the safety testing to be integrated into

the normal hospital procedures without employing specialized personnel.
Testing in this manner, however, requires supervision by skilled personnel,
who must confirm by periodic sample testing with more precise instruments
that the GO, NO-GO indications are indeed valid. Skilled personnel are also
needed for the other phase of testing, initial testing of new or altered
installations.

The cornerstone of an effective test program is a good plan and a good
set of records. Records in testing provide an initial baseline of measurements
against which later readings may be compared, a log showing when the
test was last performed, who performed it, and the future schedule of
testing. Records tend to disappear into file cabinets, where they are ineffective unless the system includes reminders and supervision. A good
reminder in popular use is a sticker attached to each instrument, which
lists the next scheduled date for a safety check. Then, if the test is not
performed as planned, the equipment user will be in a position to call
attention to the oversight. This approach uses checks and balances to
avoid accidental neglect and may, in the process, prevent accidents. There
must, in addition, be a supervisor whose primary function is to contribute
the discipline needed if effective safety testing is to be achieved. He scans
the test records and provides all the necessary directions for safety-test
personnel.

A comprehensive safety-test program of an installation consists of tests
for ground integrity, proper power distribution, and leakage.

Ground Testing

The objective of ground testing is to ensure that ground resistance is
small enough that leakage and fault currents in the ground leads are
unlikely to harm personnel nearby. The ground is tested by injecting a
known current and measuring the voltage drop across the ground conductor. Ground resistance is then calculated as the ratio of voltage to
current.

The process of taking two distinct measurements, voltage and current,
can be avoided by a resistance-measuring instrument using a voltmeter
calibrated directly in terms of resistance. Since voltage and resistance
correspond only at one value of current, accurate adjustment of current
is essential to the functioning of this instrument. One way to do this is to
provide a calibrating control R_1 (Fig. 6-1b) and a fixed calibrating resistance
R_2. During calibration, the two test leads are held together, causing all
current to flow via R_2. If the meter scale does not then indicate the numeric

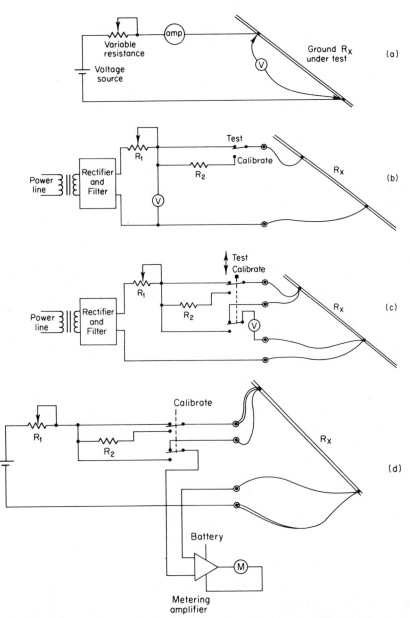

Fig. 6-1 Ground-resistance measurement. (A) The basic technique sends a known current through the path to be measured and reads the voltage drop. (b) Meter calibration can be maintained despite power-source variations by using calibrating resistance R_2 to adjust R_1. (c) The high-current technique gains sufficient voltage drop by utilizing a large current during measurement. (d) The low-current technique requires amplification of the measured voltage for adequate meter deflection.

value of R_2, the test current is not properly set and R_1 is readjusted for coincidence. The instrument then reads resistance correctly.

The ground-resistance values to be measured are quite small, ranging from 5 to several hundred milliohms. To obtain usable meter deflections, either a substantial current must be injected into the ground or the voltage drop must first be amplified before metering. Both methods have advantages and disadvantages.

The first method, using a large current, is recommended by the National Fire Protection Association (NFPA No. 70) for the measurement of ESPA ground integrity. It requires enough power so that the use of batteries becomes impractical, and the injection current of approximately 20 amp is inherently hazardous to patients in the vicinity of the ground. Thus, this method must not be used in ESPA while the area is in use.

One implementation of the high-current method is shown in Fig. 6-1c, in which a low-voltage, high-current transformer is used to supply the current via a rheostat R_1. The ac currents are rectified into dc and filtered, and are then applied to the ground to be tested. The device has four terminals, two for currents and two for voltages. Since the resistance being measured may be very small, the presence of any additional lead resistance might cause a reading error unless metering is done directly across the ground to be measured. By connecting the voltage leads directly to the ground, an accurate reading is obtained even when there is a significant voltage drop in the current leads. The circuit in Fig. 6-1c also provides means for calibrating a resistance meter as already described; because of the 4-terminal arrangement, the meter is switched so that it reads the voltage across not only R_2 but also the metering leads. The high-current method does not ensure that the ground resistance as measured with a large current is equal to the resistance obtained with small currents because the large current may temporarily overcome otherwise poor surface-to-surface contacts (Chapter 4).

In the low-current method (Fig. 6-1d), the current may be small enough to permit batteries to be used for instrument power (10–100 mA), but the measured voltages will only be in the microvolt region. Electronic amplification will therefore be necessary to attain the milliamperes required for adequate meter deflection. The low-current method is much more susceptible to interference from other small stray currents in the ground than the high-current method. Thus, confusing and sometimes erroneous measurements are not uncommon. More sophisticated instruments may be used to counteract such interference. These make use of test waveforms other than dc or power-line ac and employ filters to reject common interference signals before metering.

Area Resistance Measurements

Measuring the resistance of surface areas such as hospital flooring is slightly more complex than simple point-to-point resistance measurements because the particular path taken by the current determines the electrical resistance. In wire conductors, at least at power-line frequencies, all the current is channelled uniformly through the conductor so that current distribution is not important. This may no longer be true when current flows across a wide area, causing contact size, shape, and location to affect the resistance measurement.

In order to obtain uniform test results, the resistance of a given material is specified in terms of current flowing uniformly throughout the material.

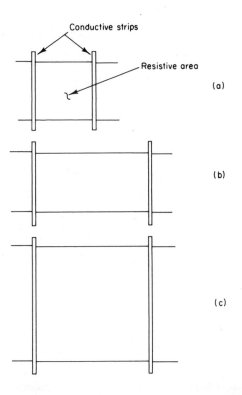

Fig. 6-2   Resistance of surface areas. When the resistance between the two end strips is measured in (b), it will read twice the resistance of (a), since length was doubled. To reduce resistance to the value measured in (a), width must be doubled as in (c). This shows that squares of whatever size have same resistance when same material is used.

In practice, this is accomplished by using conductive bars of length L, which are placed on the material during the measurements. Two such bars, held parallel, permit material resistance to be determined.

The measurements on surfaces are in reality volume measurements made across a surface having a finite thickness. The thickness affects its resistance, and more thickness decreases surface resistance. Thus, for flooring, one can expect the abrasion from constant wear to decrease the floor thickness gradually, leading to increased resistance.

Area resistance is measured in ohms per square. This odd terminology may be understood by a reference to Fig. 6-2 where a measurement is illustrated across a resistive area using two parallel conducting strips. When spacing is such that the strip spacing in Fig. 6-2b is twice that of Fig. 6-2a,

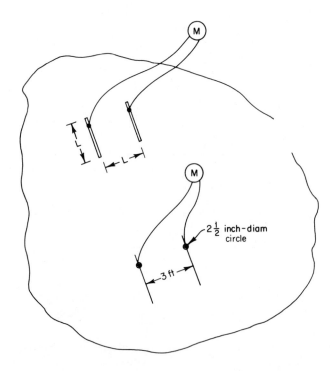

Fig. 6-3   Area resistance measurements such as on partially conductive flooring. The general technique uses conductive blocks of any length L to measure resistance. The resistance per square is obtained when the two blocks are parallel and spaced by distance L. A standardized measurement for hospital operating-room floors specifies the shape and spacing of the measurement electrodes, as well as the force to be exerted during measurement.

twice the resistance is obtained. When, however, the area width is doubled, a measurement over the same length as in Fig. 6-2b yields again the resistance value of Fig. 6-2a. Thus, the areas in Figs. 6-2c and 6-2a have the same resistance. In fact, the measured resistance will be the same for all squares, no matter what their sizes, which leads to the unit of measurement of resistance per square. Resistance of operating room floors range from 2000 to 80,000 ohms per square.

Resistance per square is measured using two parallel bars of any length L, connected to an ohmmeter, as shown in Fig. 6-3. A valid reading is obtained when the conductive bars are held parallel, are spaced exactly distance L apart, and pressure is applied on the bars to ensure good contact. Other, more specialized measurements may be utilized. Thus, for example, the hospital-floor measuring technique recommended by the National Fire Protection Association (NFPA No. 56A) suggests the use of two circular electrodes $2\frac{1}{2}$ in. in diameter and spaced 3 ft apart, applied with a force of at least 5 lb. The required floor resistance then lies between 25,000 ohms and 1 megohm. These results cannot be readily related to ohms per square.

Area measurements are made by methods described earlier, using injected current and determining voltage drops but, because resistances are generally larger, larger voltages than those for measuring wire resistance must be available from the test instrument. A 500-V source is recommended by NFPA, having a sufficiently large internal impedance so that no more than 5 mA can flow upon short circuit. This permits metering currents in the range of 500 μA to 4 mA, amounts adequate for satisfactory meter deflections.

Power-Distribution Testing

The installation of a power-distribution system is normally performed by a contractor under supervision of professional architects or engineers. Renovations and alterations, on the other hand, might be performed by the maintenance staff. All these activities involve some testing, but seldom include the type of testing necessary to ensure a safe patient environment. It is thus necessary to augment any prior testing by the following additional tests.

A. *Polarization testing* to ensure that the receptacles are properly connected to the power lines and grounds;

B. *Neutral-to-ground testing* to ensure that both are grounded and that they are not reversed;

C.   *Line voltage testing* to determine voltage differences among power receptacles;

D.   *Receptacle-force testing* to ensure that the contact between plugs and sockets is adequate.

A.   *Polarization Testing*

Power receptacles must be connected properly and uniformly so that an instrument may be plugged into any outlet (of the same kind) without adverse consequences. In a grounded distribution system (in contrast with ungrounded systems such as 230-V lines and isolated power systems), every acceptable power receptacle has three terminals—the ungrounded (hot) terminal, the neutral power return, and the safety U-ground.

Measurements can be made among these three terminals to ascertain whether proper polarization exists and to detect abnormal conditions. Six fault conditions are possible among three terminals: any of the three leads might be open, and three ways of interchanging connections exist. (This assumes that only one fault occurs at a time.) The normal receptacle arrangement is shown in Fig. 6-4, along with the three voltage measurements to be made. The fault may be uniquely deduced from measurements

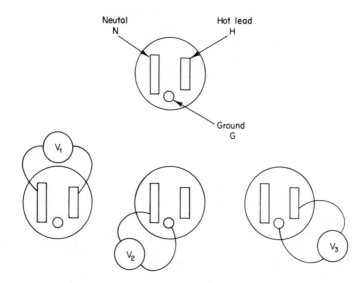

Fig. 6-4   Connecting faults in receptacles. Six likely faults are H, N, or G not connected, and H–N, H–G, or N–G reverse-connected. Of the six likely faults, five can be determined by taking the three voltmeter measurements shown. Reversal of N and G cannot be distinguished from a "good" measurement.

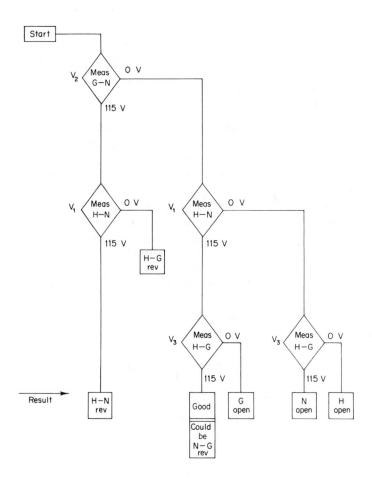

Fig. 6-5 Polarity measurement on 3-wire receptacle. Key: H, hot line; N, neutral; G, ground. Open wires and interchanges can be detected, except G–N interchange.

V_1, V_2, and V_3 with one exception—the reversal of neutral with U-ground. Figure 6-5 shows how the conclusions are drawn. In a 115-V system, first reading V_2: when $V_2 = 115$ V a fault is indicated, which is isolated by observing V_1. If $V_1 = 115$ V, the hot and neutral leads are reversed, whereas if $V_1 = 0$ V, the hot and U-ground are reversed. Similarly when $V_2 = 0$ V and $V_1 = 115$ V, one must also observe V_3 before a unique fault determination can be made. When $V_3 = 115$ V, no fault is present but an undetectable reversal of neutral with U-ground is still possible. On the other hand, when $V_3 = 0$, the U-ground is open. Following the path to the far right, when $V_1 = 0$ V and $V_3 = 0$ V, the hot lead is open.

Instead of using a voltmeter and taking three measurements, a set of three lamps could be used, each rated at power-line voltage. These lamps replace V_1, V_2, and V_3. The lamp patterns shown in Fig. 6-6 determine the fault condition. Note again that the indication for "Good" is identical with that for "Reversed G–N," which makes these two conditions indistinguishable.

Even more convenient are instruments from which the type of fault can be read directly. One such device uses a voltmeter having its meter scale subdivided into several regions, each representing a unique fault. Instead of the numeric voltmeter scale, the actual fault type is engraved onto the scale. The deflection of the needle into one or another of these regions thus permits direct readout of faults to take place. Such instruments are commercially available. They use circuits similar to those shown in Fig. 6-7a, wherein the values of the components are carefully chosen so that each fault causes the meter to deflect only into its designated scale region. The voltage registered on the voltmeter depends upon the current through R_1, which in turn varies according to which contacts of the electrical plug are at the same potential. In a properly connected power system, both the neutral and the U-ground are at the same voltage, as shown in Fig. 6-7b, so that R_2 and R_3 act in parallel, but under other than normal conditions, the resistances R_1, R_2, and R_3 combine in other ways, and the meter deflects differently. A more detailed analysis of this circuit is given in Appendix I.

Condition	V_1	V_2	V_3
Normal	●	○	●
Open H	○	○	○
Open N	○	○	●
Open G	●	○	○
Reversed H N	●	●	○
Reversed H G	○	●	●
Reversed G N	●	○	●

Shaded — on

Fig. 6-6   Indications obtained for normal and fault conditions using 3-measurement method.

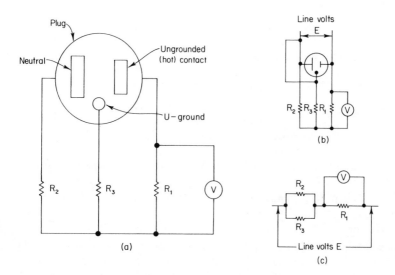

Fig. 6-7 Direct-reading receptacle-fault indicator. (a) Typical circuit. (b) Same circuit showing interconnection into properly wired power system. (c) Rearranged version of circuit in (b).

B. *Neutral-to-Ground Testing*

The receptacle testing discussed earlier fails to distinguish reversals of the neutral-to-ground connections from properly wired receptacles. Thus, there is a need for another measurement to guard against this reversal. Neutral-to-ground tests are difficult to perform because the wire resistance is not very predictable, because current flow due to biomedical instruments may be present, and because small dc currents in the neutral lead can cause erroneous meter indications. Biomedical instruments may sometimes be disconnected during the tests, and this helps considerably. When this is not possible, the influence of other instruments may in part be reduced by applying an artificial test load having a current drain far in excess of that of all other instruments. A 10-amp load often serves this purpose.

Dc current components in the neutral lead may be due to transformer imbalances or may be introduced by equipments connected to the power lines. Meters reacting only to ac components do not sense these dc components. Frequently, however, dc meter movements are used in conjunction with bridge rectifiers for neutral-to-ground testing, and these devices react to both dc and ac.* The meter indication then represents 1.11 times

---

* All combination ac/dc instruments fall into this category; an instrument that measures only ac could employ an ac or a dc meter movement, and identification must be made from manufacturer's information.

the dc component plus the effective (rms) ac component. Using switches, the bridge rectifier may be disconnected during measurements, and the same meter movement can then measure only the dc component. Having both measurements permits the ac component to be computed using the relationship

$$V_{ac} = V_{ind} - 1.11 \times V_{dc}$$

where V_{ind} is the reading with rectifiers, V_{dc} the reading without rectifiers, and V_{ac} the ac component only (see Appendix A).

A technique for measuring neutral-to-ground voltages is shown in Fig. 6-8, in which the voltage drop caused by equipment current flow is measured. When the receptacles are properly connected, all the equipment currents flow via only the hot and neutral conductors. The U-ground conductor carries at most a small leakage current. Then, when voltage-drop measurements are made with respect to a common ground reference, the voltage V_1 is usually much larger than V_2 because of the much larger current in the neutral conductor. In a properly connected system, dc components and currents from other equipments flow through the neutral rather than the U-ground lead, and this lead is therefore subject to more

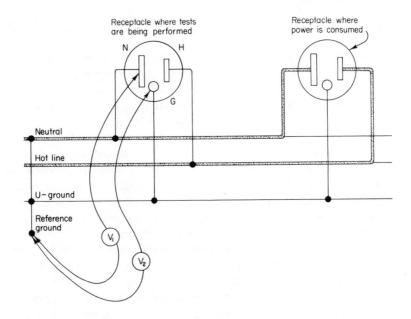

Fig. 6-8 Neutral and U-ground measurements. Different voltage drops V_1 and V_2 are due to the large differences in currents flowing in neutral versus U-ground.

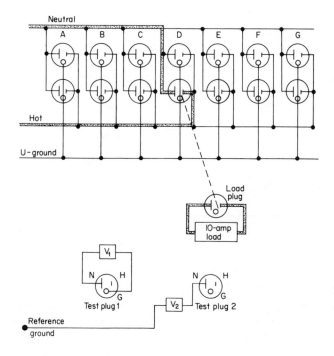

Fig. 6-9 String measurement technique showing current flow (heavy lines) when a 10-amp test load is plugged into D. Test plugs 1 or 2 are then plugged alternately into each receptacle.

amplitude changes and noise. When V_2 is observed to be noisy or to vary considerably, reversals of the ground-to-neutral leads should be suspected.

Another technique uses string measurements as shown in Fig. 6-9 to check for proper neutral-to-ground connections. This figure depicts a series of wall receptacles connected together by conventional electric wiring. A small amount of resistance is present in each wire lead, which is used to detect voltage drops. A 10-amp load is wired to a plug, and this load may be connected to one of the wall receptacles. The metering voltmeters are also wired to plugs; two alternates are given. The first method shows V_1 measured between the neutral and ground connection on the plug; it is used to measure neutral-to-ground voltage at each receptacle. With a 10-amp flow in the neutral lead from the receptacle into which the load was plugged toward the power source, the voltage V_1 will progressively decrease at each receptacle as the power source is approached. Very little, if any, current flows in the U-ground lead, so that the total measurement reflects the voltage drop in the neutral conductors. When the load is

Table 6-1
Decision Process in String Measuring Technique

System wiring	Test voltage	Load plugged into	Test plug into A	B	C	D	E	F	G
Proper	V_1 or V_2	D	Decreasing voltage ←			Same voltage			
	V_1 or V_2	F	Decreasing voltage ←					Same voltage	
Reversed GN at D	V_1	D	Same as first line						
	V_2	D	Zero			Voltage reading		Zero	

plugged into receptacle D, for example, the voltmeter indication decreases as the voltmeter is plugged, in turn, into C, B, and A. On the other hand, since no current flows in the lines linking D, E, F, and G, no voltage drop occurs in these lines and the V_1 readings for D, E, F, and G are identical.*

Suppose, instead of being wired properly, the ground and neutral leads were reversed at receptacle D. The current now travels via U-ground rather than the neutral conductor. Because of the way in which V_1 is wired, the same value of V_1 will register and the fault will not be detected. By using the second of the two alternate plug wiring connections, this ambiguity is avoided. A plug is again used, but only one connection of the voltmeter is now made, to the neutral conductor. The second connection is routed externally to the reference ground. In a properly wired system, the readings V_1 and V_2 are identical. But when a neutral-to-ground reversal is present, the readings will differ. In the receptacle location where the reversal has occurred, V_1 and V_2 are still the same, but at all other receptacles, V_2 falls to zero. Table 6-1 summarizes the results obtained with the string measurement method.

Neutral-to-ground resistance can also be measured, but the measurements are subject to the same difficulties previously described for voltage tests; hence, unambiguous results are also difficult to obtain. Sophisticated techniques can circumvent the disadvantages. For example, the test current from the ohmmeter might have signal and frequency characteristics quite different from those of the interference, which makes it possible to use frequency filters within the metering circuits to discriminate against undesirable signals. Such ohmmeters, however, are complex and are not generally available.

* It is assumed here that all other biomedical instrumentation has been disconnected.

C. Line-Voltage Testing

Line-voltage tests are performed by measuring the ac voltages between all the ungrounded, hot terminals in a specific locale. The reasons for possible differences in line voltages were described in Chapter 4, where it was shown that in a typical distribution system, the voltages from one ungrounded terminal to another may be identical or may differ by 115, 200, or 230 V (Fig. 4-10). An ac voltmeter measurement among all receptacles readily establishes whether any such voltage differences exist in a given installation. The most desirable condition, in which electricity is supplied from the same power-line phase and distribution line, is indicated by a measurement of zero volts between corresponding points of different receptacles.

D. Receptacle-Force Testing

A plug inserted into a wall socket establishes electrical contact by the insertion of a rigid blade into a spring-loaded metal contact. As long as the spring retains adequate clamping force, good contact is made. But with aging, and often as a result of arcing in the receptacle, the springiness of the material weakens, finally resulting in poor contact and possible danger to personnel.

The quality of the contact can be assessed by measuring the amount of force it takes to remove the plug from the receptacle. This force is the aggregate of the retention forces on each separate metallic contact and may include other force contributions resulting from misalignments. The best measure of electrical contact quality is obtained by separately measuring the extracting force from each contact. This is done by using a calibrated spring or similar instrument, from which the amount of force can be directly read.

Although the minimum allowable force is specified by industry standards, these do not take into account the additional safety factors needed in health-care facilities and do not make allowances for wear. Good and relatively new springs result in tension forces well above 1 lb; such contacts are tight to the feel of personnel involved in plugging and unplugging equipment. Old and worn receptacles, on the other hand, often have springs measuring less than 8 oz. In practice, the lower limit is best placed at 10 oz per contact. When tension falls below this limit, excessive wear is indicated and the receptacle should be replaced.

Testing for receptacle force presents a good opportunity to also conduct a visual inspection of the receptacle for signs of burning, chipping, or breakage, all of which are early signs of possible health hazards.

Electrical Leakage

Electrical leakage represents extraneous current flow along paths other than those intended. In the context of this book, electrical leakage means extraneous currents in or out of grounds and other patient-connected leads. Although patient leads are usually confined to the vicinity of the patient and are not usually connected to other persons or into other rooms, the grounds associated with these patient leads may have metallic continuity throughout the building and even outside the health-care facility. They can thereby carry leakage currents from one locale to another.

Leakage currents may be continuous or intermittent, and they may originate by direct connection, by capacitive coupling, or by radiation. The mere existence of a leakage current may not necessarily present a hazard to personnel, but when such a current is sufficiently large in magnitude, of unfavorable waveshape, and applied to electrically susceptible patients, serious health hazards can result. By far the most common source of electrical leakage in ESPA's is power-line ac flowing either in the ground or in a patient lead. In a properly arranged installation, these leakage currents can originate only in the instruments used at the immediate location, other leakage currents having been previously detoured away from the site by proper grounding.

Leakage originating in an instrument may be incidental to its design, or it may be due to a fault in the instrument. There are three principal sources for incidental leakage: the line cords, the power-line filters, and the power transformer. All these leakages are capacitive in nature and occur because ac is used for power.

A. *Line Cords*

The close proximity of the two power leads in the line cord causes stray electric current to flow from one power lead to the other along the entire length of the line cord. The leakage current varies both with length and with the choice of insulating material. At 120 V, 60 Hz, the leakage current is

$$I \text{ (microamperes/foot)} = 0.0452 \times C \text{ (picofarads/foot)}$$

The capacitance varies over a relatively narrow range, so that the leakage current generally ranges between 1.4 and 2.3 μA/ft in commercially available line cords. Proper grounding can divert this current away from the patient. In conventional electrical branch wiring, where one power conductor (the neutral) is grounded, line-cord leakage currents are diverted from the site via the neutral conductor. But a third wire, the U-ground, is also present in the line cord, which allows leakage currents to flow into the ground at the patient site. When an isolated power system is used, both power leads are ungrounded. Although the same leakage still occurs between the power conductors, leakage current will not flow into the ground unless the isolated power system is seriously unbalanced. This is true even in the presence of the U-ground conductor, because in a balanced system, the amount of leakage current flowing from one power line into the U-ground conductor is returned from the U-ground to the other power conductor.

B. *Power-Line Filters*

Some equipments use capacitors or combinations of inductors and capacitors connected from the power lines to ground to remove undesirable spurious signals generated within the equipment. Other equipments may employ capacitors for power-factor correction. Although these capacitors may be necessary to meet certain regulatory requirements, they channel extraneous leakage currents into the grounds. The leakage current is proportional to the capacitance used, and the leakage due to filters is often larger than that contributed by line cords. Thus, from a safety point of view, line filters are very undesirable in biomedical instruments. At 120 V, 60 Hz, the leakage current is

$$I \text{ (microamperes)} = 0.0452 \times C \text{ (picofarads)}$$

C. *Transformer Capacitance*

The power transformer of an instrument accepts the power-line voltage into the primary winding and distributes power from its secondary winding. Both windings are placed on a metallic core of material suitable for the transfer of the energy between the windings. The proximity of the primary winding to the core and to the secondary winding causes leakage currents to flow among the windings and to the core. These are capacitive in nature and exist in addition to the normal inductive coupling necessary for power transfer. Electrostatic shields are often placed between the windings and sometimes between windings and core, and these shields can be made to reduce the leakage currents into grounds. Of particular interest is the leakage current from the primary winding to ground, which varies considerably among instruments, depending upon the physical size of the transformer, how it is constructed, and which side of the primary winding happens to be connected to the neutral conductor. Capacitances range typically from 5 to 300 pF, causing leakage currents up to 14 μA per instrument.

Instrument-Leakage Testing

Electrical leakage in instruments may occur in many ways, and a test program must make allowances for all possibilities. To ensure that testing is indeed comprehensive, leakage measurements must be conducted from and into every terminal that might conceivably be involved in contact with the patient. The terminals to be considered are the power leads (1, 2), the U-ground (3), the outer case of the equipment (4), and the signal leads (5, 6, etc.). The signal leads, which include the patient leads, may occur in pairs, in which case they are designated 5A, 5B, 6A, 6B, etc. Although leakage may be present from any terminal to any other, significant current flow is likely in only a few, and these will be described further. In any case, for a specific instrument, every important path must be recognized and its electrical leakage tested.

The terminals of a typical instrument with two pairs of patient terminals are shown in Fig. 6-10a. The power-input terminals are usually arranged in one of the two ways shown in Figs. 6-10b and 6-10c. The more common version (Fig. 6-10b) uses a single ground system, and the U-ground from the line cord is tied to case ground. The transformer core, having been mounted on the chassis, is also grounded to the case. The arrangement in Fig. 6-10c, on the other hand, is used where special effort has been made to reduce leakage currents. It uses electrostatic shields in the transformer to reduce interwinding capacitance. The primary-winding shield is connected to the U-ground, which, however, is not otherwise connected within the instrument. The transformer core and the secondary-winding shield are connected to chassis ground. When the instrument case is metallic, the chassis is in electrical contact with the outer case but when the outer case is fully insulated, there is no such electrical contact. Point 4 in the figure represents the outer case. When insulated, only small capacitive currents can still flow through the case. Leakage measurements are still necessary, using an artificial metallic surface attached to the outer case. By convention, this test surface is to be a piece of foil 10 × 20 cm.

Comparing Fig. 6-10b with Fig. 6-10c, note that because 3 and 4 are electrically equivalent in Fig. 6-10b, leakage measurements out of 4 can be made meaningful only by first disconnecting all the leads into 3. For this reason, a procedure suitable for a variety of different instruments

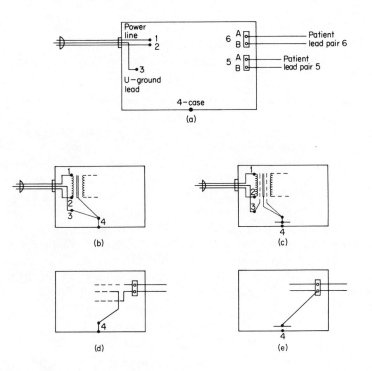

Fig. 6-10 Instrument input/output terminals. (a) Critical leakage terminals. (b) Conventional grounded three-wire system. (c) Double-insulated power input. (d) Balanced, ungrounded patient leads. (e) Single-ended patient leads.

should include provisions for disconnecting the U-ground lead during some measurements.

The relationships of the patient-lead configurations with ground are shown in Figs. 6-10d and 6-10e. The balanced or double-ended pair in Fig. 6-10d normally has a high impedance to ground for patient protection. The connection in Fig. 6-10e is single-ended and has one terminal tied to the chassis. In conventional input circuits as in Fig. 6-10b, an undesirable low-impedance path from the patient to ground is thereby provided. Newer equipments avoid this configuration.

The four common leakage paths relevant to patient safety are shown in Fig. 6-11. These are

1. the power-line leakages to case and U-ground, from 1, 2 to 3, 4;
2. the power-line leakages to patient leads, from 1, 2 to 5, 6;

3.   the leakages among patient leads contributed by power from inside the equipment, which appear among 5 and 6;

4.   the leakage paths from patient leads to case, from 5, 6 to 4 and from 4 to 5, 6.

Each case will be discussed further, and measurement sequences will be described.

Suitable measuring instruments must be capable of indicating all currents that might be hazardous to patients. Experiments with dogs have indicated that the tolerable limits tend to increase with the applied ac frequency. One way to conduct the measurement consists of compensating the measuring device so that the higher and less dangerous frequencies result in smaller meter indications. In this way, the indication more truly represents the hazard. Such compensation is shown in Fig. 6-12, where the response shown in the curve is obtained by shunting the 500-ohm resistance by a resistance–capacitance combination. At progressively higher frequencies, the resistance across which measurements are made is then reduced to as small a value as 2.55 ohms because the capacitor allows

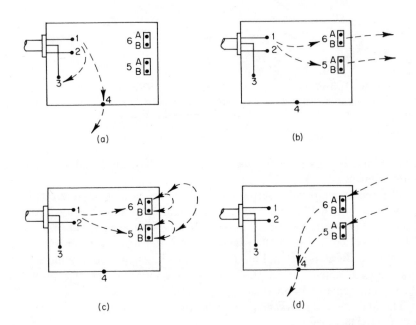

Fig. 6-11 Four common leakage paths in instruments. (a) From power lines into U-ground and case. (b) From power lines into patient terminals. (c) Among patient terminals. (d) From internal or external sources via patient terminals to ground.

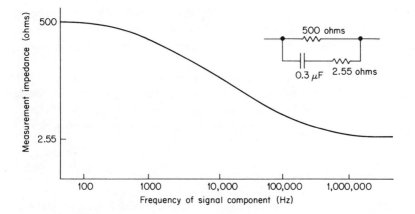

Fig. 6-12 Response of a variable-impedance measurement circuit, which compensates frequency response to hazard.

progressively more current to flow through the 2.55-ohm resistance. The curve is intended to match the experimental findings made with dogs.

When measurements need to be made across a resistance other than 500 ohms, the bypass resistance and capacitance assume different values as follows:*

bypass resistance = 5.11/1000 × metering impedance (ohms)

capacitance = 150/metering impedance (microfarads)

A second factor affecting meter indication and hazards is the presence of dc with ac. Again, it is known that the hazards due to ac are more serious than those due to dc, and regulatory limits for ac are frequently tighter. Thus, separation of measurements into ac and dc components is desirable. The most commonly used metering scheme makes use of a dc meter movement with a bridge rectifier to which a combination of ac and dc can be applied. This arrangement responds to all hazards, either ac or dc, but it does not respond equally to both. The error, however, is not large. In the conventional arrangement, the meter is calibrated using a pure sine wave,

* These formulations apply to measurements where a low-impedance path exists to the patient's heart. The compensation curve and bypass resistance differ for other health-care instrumentation, as follows:

The limit of 500 μA up to 1000 Hz rises to 10 mA at 100 kHz; the capacitance remains unchanged, but the bypass resistance becomes

bypass resistance = 52.3/1000 × metering impedance (ohms)

and the meter scale shows the effective (rms) value of the sine wave. Actually, the meter movement does not sense the effective value, but only the average of the ac–dc combination. The net result is an 11% error in indication when pure dc is applied.

Ac and dc may be separated by switching as in Fig. 6-13. When on dc, currents flow directly through the meter movement, bypassing the bridge rectifier. The meter is then insensitive to the ac components and measures only the dc component. The computation for the ac component is given in Appendix A.

A.   *Power-Line Leakage to Case*

Leakage from power lines depends upon the internal instrument arrangement as well as the power distribution system. Figure 6-14 illustrates this point. A conventional power system supplies power to the instrument in Fig. 6-14a. This power system has a grounded neutral conductor so that terminals 2 and 3 are in fact at the same potential. When the instrument has only a single ground, terminal 4 is also tied to this combination. Leakage can then occur from terminal 1 only, via any number of internal paths to grounds 2, 3, and 4. Terminal 2, however, is grounded only at a faraway point, and any leakage into this point will not appear at 3 and 4 and cannot therefore contribute leakage currents into the local ground. The dashed lines show the leakage path. The same conventional power distribution system is shown in Fig. 6-14b, along with the leakage path

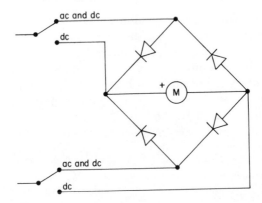

Fig. 6-13   Bridge method of using a dc meter for ac and dc measurements. In the "ac and dc" position, the meter reads the average value of the combined voltages. When the meter scale is calibrated to read the rms value of pure sine-wave ac, dc components are 11% in error. In the dc position, the meter reads only the dc component.

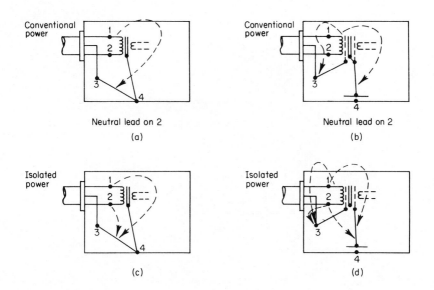

Fig. 6-14 Dependence of power-line leakage upon distribution system and internal grounding. In branch circuits where a neutral lead is at ground potential, leakage occurs from the hot wire to ground. (a) Conventional instruments have the U-ground tied to the case so that leakage currents divide among 3 and 4. (b) In double-grounded systems, case 4 is separated from U-ground 3. Because of shielding, leakage to 4 is minimized. Similar conditions prevail for isolated power systems (c) and (d), but leakage originates in each power line.

for a double-grounded instrument. Again, terminal 2 cannot contribute to leakage current. With 3 and 4 separated, and because of shielding, most leakage will channel via 3, which conducts it harmlessly via the U-ground of the power cord. Only a small leakage component flows through terminal 4. The leakage paths for the same instruments, connected to an isolated power system, are shown in Figs. 6-14c and 6-14d. Since neither power line is grounded, leakage can be expected from both terminals 1 and 2. In Fig. 6-14c, these leakage currents channel into the combination of grounds 3 and 4, whereas in Fig. 6-14d they divide among 3 and 4, with very little leakage appearing on 4.

Leakage measurements are made by inserting a meter into the ground lead. The point with worst potential hazard, terminal 4 (case), is selected. Under normal conditions, 3 is grounded via the U-ground. When points 3 and 4 are internally connected, the leakage measurement out of 4 is shunted by the connection through the U-ground. This helps to protect the patient. In the eventuality that a wire break occurs in the U-ground, all the leakage current flows via 4. This condition is measured by opening

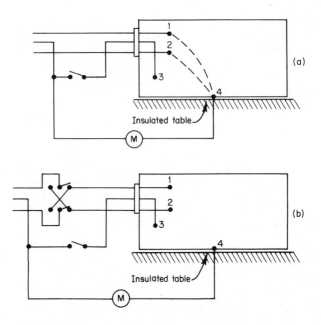

Fig. 6-15 Power-line leakage measurement. (a) By disconnecting the U-ground, all leakage currents are diverted via the case. Measurement with a meter then gives the worst-case exposure. (b) To allow for the possibility that leakage might be worse when power lines are accidentally reversed, a measurement is taken with power both normal and reversed.

the U-ground lead temporarily. Figure 6-15a shows a test arrangement that is easily obtained by inserting a test fixture between power lines and instrument. In order to account for abnormal but not unlikely situations, leakage is also measured with the power-line leads reversed, as in Fig. 6-15b, using a reversing switch. This test will reveal which connection of the transformer leads results in minimum current leakage. Both conditions (a) and (b) are tested with the instrument power switch both on and off because at times the leakage current with power off can be larger than that with power on. Table 6-2 shows the eight measurements necessary for a complete appraisal of power-line leakage conditions. By performing all these measurements, it is unnecessary to be cognizant of the internal circuit configurations used in a particular instrument. The maximum reading reveals the worst potential hazard condition.

Absolute leakage current limits are in process of being established by a number of regulatory agencies, and some limits now under consideration are listed in Table 6-3. A distinction is generally made between the con-

Table 6-2
Power-Line Leakage Measurements

Test	Power	U-ground lead	Power connection
A1	Off	Closed	Normal
A2			Reversed
A3		Open	Normal
A4			Reversed
A5	On	Closed	Normal
A6			Reversed
A7		Open	Normal
A8			Reversed

ditions under which the equipment is to be utilized, the most stringent limits being proposed for sites where a low-impedance path to the patient's heart is likely to exist.

B. *Power-Line Leakage to Patient Leads*

Measurement of power-line leakage to patient leads is made by monitoring the current flow out of the patient lead into ground. Figure 6-16a shows the arrangement, which includes provisions for opening the U-ground and for reversal of input power. Two measurements are required for each pair of patient leads, so that this test may be quite lengthy. Testing may be simplified by connecting all the patient leads together and measuring the total leakage current due to all leads. When the results show excessive leakage current, individual measurements may then be made to isolate the leakage source. The arrangement for simultaneous testing is shown in Fig. 6.16b. This measurement should also be made on instruments with

Table 6-3
Regulatory Limits for Power-Line Leakage[a]

	NFPA 76 BM	California AHA	UL 544
Low-impedance			
path to patient	100 ac	10 rms	10 ac
heart	100 dc		14 dc
In other patient	500 ac	500 rms	100 ac
areas	500 dc		140 dc

[a] All values in microamperes.

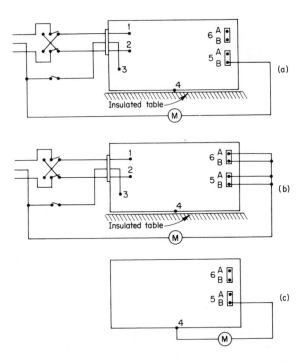

Fig. 6-16 Power leakage into patient leads. Connections for externally powered equipments are shown in (a). Measurements are made to each patient lead in turn. The simplified technique in (b) measures all patient leads simultaneously. For self-powered instruments, measurement is made as in (c). Again, all patient leads can be measured simultaneously (not shown).

self-contained power sources, as in Fig. 6-16c, because excessive leakage currents cannot even then be precluded.

The eight tests in Table 6-2 are again required, but they are repeated N times for N patient terminals, as shown in Table 6-4, or just once when simultaneous measurements reveal acceptable leakage currents. For self-powered equipments, only two measurements are required per patient terminal, as shown at the bottom.

The proposed leakage-current limits, which are more stringent than those involving power leakage to ground, are given in Table 6-5.

C.   *Leakage between Patient Leads*

Another potential hazard can exist from one patient lead to another. To ensure safe conditions, measurements are required from each patient lead

Table 6-4
Power-Line to Patient-Lead Leakage Measurements

Patient lead	Test	Power	U-ground lead	Power connection
5A	B1	Off	Closed	Normal
5A	B2			Reversed
⋮	⋮			
5B	B1	Off	Closed	Normal
5B	B2			Reversed
⋮	⋮			
8B	B5	On	Closed	Normal
8B	B6			Reversed
8B	B7		Open	Normal
8B	B8			Reversed

Tests for self-powered instruments

5A	B1	Off
5A	B2	On
5B	B1	Off
⋮	⋮	

Table 6-5
Regulatory Limits for Power-Line to Patient-Lead Leakage[a]

	NFPA 76 BM	California AHA	UL 544	VA X1414	AAMI
Low-impedance path to patient heart	10 ac 50 dc	10 rms	5 ac 7 dc	10 rms	10 rms, 200 peak-to-peak pulse or transient decaying to 28 peak-to-peak within 5 msec
In other patient areas	50 ac 250 dc	10 rms	50 ac 70 dc		500 rms

[a] All values in microamperes.

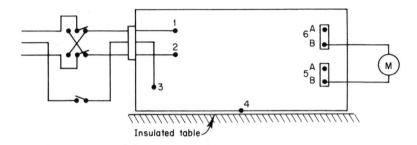

Fig. 6-17   Leakage among patient leads. A test is conducted from each patient lead to all others. When there are N patient terminals $N(N - 1)/2$ complete sets of measurements are required.

to all others. Figure 6-17 shows how such a measurement is made. Since simultaneous measurements are not possible, the number of measurements required increases very rapidly as the number of patient terminals increases. For N patient leads, $N \times (N - 1)/2$ complete sets of readings are made, each set consisting of the same eight readings already described. The proposed leakage-current limits are given in Table 6-6.

D. *Patient-Lead Leakage to Case*

Patient-lead leakage to case may be due to internal or external causes. When due to external causes, currents originating outside the instrument may be routed along the patient leads into the instrument and from there to ground. The internal circuitry plays an important role in protecting the patient from dangers from this source by limiting the leakage possible under these circumstances to small values. Test I is performed to check on

Table 6-6
Regulatory Limits for Interpatient-Lead Leakage[a]

	NFPA 76 BM	California AHA	UL 544
Low-impedance path to patient heart	10 ac 50 dc	10 rms	5 ac 7 dc
In other patient areas	50 ac 250 dc	10 rms	50 ac 70 dc

[a] All values in microamperes.

this potential leakage source. Danger may also be present due to patient-lead leakage currents when the case of the instrument is accidentally exposed to power-line voltages. Test II checks this condition.

In either test, an artificial current is injected by the application of power-line voltage via a protective resistance either to the patient leads or to the case. The test circuit is shown in Fig. 6-18a. During test I, the equipment is maintained in its normally grounded condition, including the grounding of the case. In test II, the grounds are disconnected and the injected current is applied to the case. Patient-lead current is monitored in each test. During the tests, personnel may be exposed to power-line voltages appearing on the instrument case or on the test device. Precautions against shock are therefore necessary during testing. The purpose of the 120,000-ohm resistance is to limit the maximum exposure of test personnel to 1 mA at 120 V. The actual current flow in ungrounded patient leads will, of course, be much smaller.

The test sequence consists of the four tests shown in Table 6-7, which embody all combinations of power on and off with normal and reversed

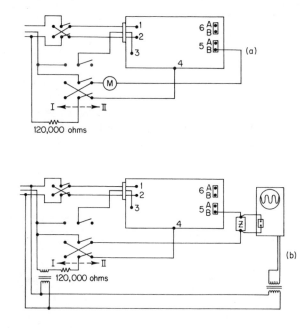

Fig. 6-18 Patient-lead injection tests. Test I: ac is applied to each patient lead in turn. Test II: ac is applied to case and U-ground is opened. Patient-lead current is monitored. (a) Basic electric circuit. (b) Additional isolation circuitry required when oscilloscope measurements are taken.

Table 6-7
Patient-Lead Injection Measurements

Test I				Test II			
Patient lead	Test	Power	Power connection	Patient lead	Test	Power	Power connection
5A	DI1	Off	Normal	5A	DII1	Off	Normal
5A	DI2		Reversed	5A	DII2		Reversed
5A	DI3	On	Normal	5A	DII3	On	Normal
5A	DI4		Reversed	5A	DII4		Reversed
5B	DI1	Off	Normal	5B	DII1	Off	Normal
5B	DI2		Reversed	5B	DII2		Reversed
⋮	⋮			⋮	⋮		

connections. The measurements are performed $2N$ times for N patient terminals, and simultaneous measurements can be made by tying all patient leads together. This test fails for grounded patient leads, as often found in older equipment, and for low-impedance patient leads. These constitute a known potential hazard when connected to patients. Table 6-8 shows the regulatory limits now being proposed for this test.

Additional precautions are necessary when line-powered test instruments such as an oscilloscope are used while testing. This action is necessary to avoid creating additional leakage paths, which might cause false readings. Figure 6-18b shows how the test circuit in Fig. 6-18a is modified by adding two isolation transformers, one for the injection current and the other for

Table 6-8
Regulatory Limits for Injected Current[a]

	NFPA 76 BM	VA X1414	AAMI
Low-impedance path to patient heart	20 ac 100 dc	10 rms	10 rms, 200 peak-to-peak pulse or transient decaying to 28 peak-to-peak within 5 msec
In other patient areas	100 ac	—	—

[a] All values in microamperes.

the line-powered test instrument. With these modifications, large pulses and other transients may be observed concurrently with leakage testing.

In summary, instrument-leakage measurements are quite extensive, involving five types of measurements. For a line-powered instrument with N patient terminals, the complete series consists of

$\quad$ 8 tests for power-line leakage to case,
$\quad$ $8N$ tests for power-line leakage to patient leads,
$8N(N - 1)/2$ tests for leakage between patient leads,
$\quad$ $8N$ tests for patient-lead leakage to case.

All measurements use the same techniques, making it practical to use commercial test instruments designed for insertion between power line and instrument. These test instruments have switches for various test conditions. Many such instruments are now available.

Installation Leakage Measurements

Leakage tests conducted on the complete installation provide aggregate results of leakage conditions among all the equipment installed at a site. The purpose of the test would in part be defeated if it involved disconnecting any equipment or leads because errors during restoration could render the measurements meaningless. For this reason, measurements in installations consist of voltage tests made across all critical points. All measurements are made with one lead connected to the patient reference grounding bus. The other lead is connected, in turn, to the ground points of all power receptacles, instrument cases and other metallic surfaces within reach of the patient. A hazardous condition is indicated whenever the voltage exceeds 5 mV, but even smaller indications often call for investigation of their origin. The measurements should be performed with all instrument power on and off, and with power applied to some instruments but not to others, so that the worst leakage condition is detected. Leakage tests to patient leads may also be made in this manner, but not while a patient occupies the site.

Most instruments will be sensitive to continuous ac and dc leakage but may well fail to detect intermittent or pulse leakage. This makes it desirable to include an occasional ground check using an oscilloscope on which unusually large nonrepetitive leakage currents can be observed. These observations, however, require skilled interpretation as to their significance with regard to safety.

Installation testing must include a check upon the continued effectiveness of the line-isolation monitor in the isolated power system. Although most monitors contain self-test features, it is desirable to conduct an independent test to verify proper operation.

In a properly isolated system and in the absence of loads connected to the system, the impedance from each power line to ground is very high. With aging, however, and under humid conditions, deterioration can take place that lowers the impedance to ground. Breakdowns, of course, can quickly do the same, and all instruments connected to the lines lower the line-to-ground impedance.

One test technique consists of measuring the impedance or resistance from line to ground with all power disconnected. A high-resistance ohmmeter can serve this purpose, providing quick indications of line-to-ground resistance. It will, however, be insensitive to capacitive leakage. The second method consists of artificially adding resistive faults until the alarm is activated and noting at which resistance value this takes place. This method is simple and does not require power disruption during testing. A comprehensive test includes simulated faults from one power line at a time to ground and simultaneous faults from both lines to ground. A test fixture for introducing artificial resistive faults can be easily constructed, as shown in Fig. 6-19.

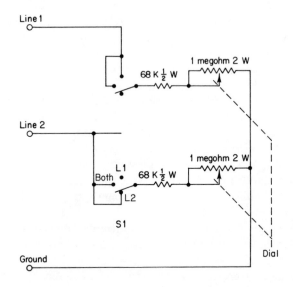

Fig. 6-19 Schematic diagram of a simple line-isolation tester. Switch S1 controls whether the simulated fault is introduced in one line, the other, or both. The adjustable control sets the fault current over a wide range. Only resistive faults are tested.

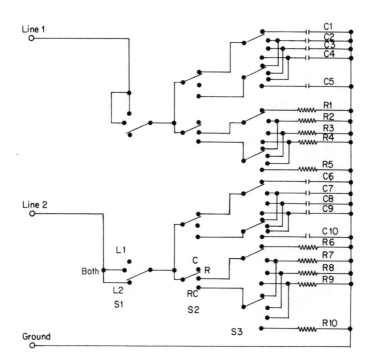

Fig. 6-20 Schematic diagram of a comprehensive line-isolation tester. Switch S1 controls whether the simulated fault is introduced in one line, the other, or both. S2 controls whether faults are resistive, capacitive, or in combination. S3 provides a selection of four values of simulated fault current.

It is not normally necessary during routine testing to introduce other than resistive faults, because the relationship, for a given monitor, between resistive and capacitive faults is fixed. This relationship may, however, become disturbed by a fault within the monitor. To include testing for this eventuality requires the introduction of capacitive as well as resistive faults. A test fixture suitable for combination testing is shown in Fig. 6-20. It contains three switches, resistances, and capacitances. Switch S1 controls whether simulated loads are applied to one power line, the other, or both. Switch S2 permits selection of resistive, capacitive, or combination faults. Switch S3 selects discrete values of resistances and capacitances. As S3 is rotated, each resistance and reactance is chosen 41% larger than the previous value, and this process reduces the total number of necessary components. For example, to simulate a fault of 120,000 ohms, either a resistance or a reactance is switched into the circuit, but when a combination resistance–capacitance of 120,000 ohms is required, the actual components have to consist of a resistance of 1.41 $\times$ 120,000 ohms and a reactance of the same value. Both are available at the next switch position.

At the present time, the maximum regulatory limit for line-current leakage in an isolated power system is set at 1 mA. Testing therefore should be conducted near this value; the corresponding impedance at 120 V is 120,000 ohms.

Bibliography

Battig, C. G., Checking for Electric Shock Hazards, *Anesthesiology* **29,** No. 5 (Sept./Oct. 1968).

Blashke, W., Automated Checking of Loop Resistance with Electronic Devices, *Angew. Elektron. Am & R* (Germany, in German) No. 6 (1971).

Collins, B., Maintenance of Medical Electronics Equipment, *Hosp. Eng. (GB)* **26** (March 1972).

Health Devices, Emergency Care Research Inst., Philadelphia, Pennsylvania.

Jordan, W. D., Standard Methods of Measuring Risk Current, *J. AAMI* **5,** No. 6 (Nov./Dec. 1971).

Lubin, D., Stringent Grounding Control, Last Minute Checks, Needed for Electrical Safety, Modern Hospital, (July 1969).

New York Univ. Med. Center Safety Manual, NYU Safety Committee.

Starmer, C. F., Whalen, R. E., and McIntosh, H. D., Determination of Leakage Currents in Medical Equipment, *Amer. J. Cardiol.* **17** (1966).

Chapter 7

ESTABLISHMENT OF A PRACTICAL SAFETY, PREVENTIVE-MAINTENANCE, AND REPAIR PROGRAM

If you have not already begun to formulate plans on how to set up a safety and preventive-maintenance program in your own hospital, then you are more than ready to read this chapter. If, however, you have a plan in mind, then you should find it worthwhile to compare your plan with the practical solution presented here.

The Need for a Safety and Maintenance Program

The need for an effective safety, maintenance, and repair program in hospitals today can be supported by many considerations, which we shall attempt to describe. Since a hospital is recognized as a place where people go to be healed and made well, then anything that is permitted to exist within this institution that can possibly cause the opposite effect could be regarded as negligence.

Safety in the hospital not only must be patient oriented, but should and must include personnel as well. A strong incentive for accomplishing a program of this type is the legal liability that could result if such a program were not established. A lawsuit brought against an institution by a claimant because he tripped and fell due to a defective floor tile is a common occurrence. The law tells the defendant that failure to maintain the floor in a safe condition is negligence. In hospitals, failure to maintain a certain "standard of care" can result in severe penalties through legal action. As a result, failure to institute and maintain a suitable scientific and medical instrumentation facility in one hospital, the responsibility of which extends to the maintenance and repair of medical equipment, while other hospitals

127

are doing so, has been regarded by the courts as contributory negligence where injury is involved. Dr. Martin Lloyd Norton, Associate Professor of Anesthesiology and Adjunct Professor of Law at Wayne State University, stated in a recent article dealing with biomedical instrumentation and liability that failure of a hospital to have a preventive maintenance program and/or use of personnel of inadequate background could be considered negligence under "reasonable man" standards. The reasonable-man concept is actually applicable to the law of torts. In a recent case (Butler versus N. W. Hospital of Minnesota), the opinion of the court stated that "The general rule is that equipment furnished by a hospital for a patient's use should be reasonably fit for the uses and purposes intended under the circumstances, and injury suffered because of failure of this duty leads to liability based on negligence."

Safety is only a word. For it to become a fact there must exist a tried and proven program of inspection, repair, and replacement. If this program also provides economic advantages, its initiation becomes even more desirable.

Hospital Size

A practical approach to initiating a workable safety and maintenance program is governed by the size of a hospital. It is evident that there is no one system that will cover hospitals of all sizes uniformly. This implies, in turn, that the size of a hospital dictates the type of program to be adopted.

The expressions "large hospital" and "small hospital" are descriptive but difficult to define nationally or world-wide. In New York State, in general, a "large hospital" could be defined as one having 400–600 beds or more, and a "small hospital" as one with 100–150 beds. A "medium-sized hospital" would consist of 150–400 beds. These definitions apply in regions that have a high population density and therefore hold true for California and other states with large urban populations.

At a recent meeting on Shared Biomedical Instrumentation Engineering Services, held in Charleston, South Carolina, one of the authors was made aware of the comparatively small size of hospitals in areas having a low population density. A representative of the Texas Hospital Association indicated that hospitals of 20–30 beds were the rule for these rural areas, rather than the exception. It is understandable that in such areas, a 100-bed institution might be considered large and, in some cases, a medical center.

A truly practical program for safety, maintenance, and repair must be flexible enough to permit expansion and contraction, so that it will essentially fit almost any hospital, regardless of its size.

There are four basic modes for accomplishing maintenance and repair of scientific and medical instrumentation within a hospital.

First, there is the call system whereby a vendor, contractor, or repair service is called whenever a piece of equipment ceases to operate or is defective. This method of accomplishing maintenance as an afterthought rather than as a preventive-maintenance program is usually very costly and offers no assurance that your equipment will be operating when you need it; in many cases it also results in loss of use of the equipment for the duration of the time required to make the necessary repairs and/or replacements.

Second, there is contract maintenance, whereby a maintenance contract is signed with an outside organization—sometimes the manufacturer, sometimes a private organization. An agreement is made, for a fee, to maintain the equipment in the hospital. Now this, too, is extremely costly because one must consider the travel time required for personnel from this organization to come to the hospital, transportation of equipment, the actual cost of labor and parts for repair, and a margin of profit for the maintenance organization.

Third, there is the shared-services program, which can be divided into two types. One is the clinical-engineering-center concept, sometimes referred to as the "central stable plan"; the other is the kingpin hospital" mode of shared biomedical instrumentation engineering.

Fourth is the straight "in-house" scientific and medical instrumentation (SMI) capability which is advisable for very large hospitals, leading institutions, and medical centers. This type of large organization usually has the money to support a completely independent department with technicians under the cognizance and control of a biomedical instrumentation engineer and is usually capable of allotting time to research and circuit development. Typical of the foregoing is Downstate Medical Center, Brooklyn, New York.

Hospitals of small size in widespread rural areas may very well depend on either the call method or a mobile-laboratory shared service such as the Clinical Engineering Center of Toledo, Ohio, offers.

Hospitals of less than 150-bed capacity, but closer to urban communities, usually turn to the second alternative of a contract for maintenance and repair, believing it is not worth the effort to initiate an SMI capability in-house. Recently however, some of these hospitals have entered the kingpin-hospital shared-engineering plan, and two hospitals that are near each other are in fact sharing a technician under the guidance and control of an engineer.

The typical suburban community hospital having usually from 150 to

300 beds is ideal for the kingpin plan and eventually winds up with an SMI laboratory manned by two in-house technicians. Control, guidance, and expert testimony, if required, are supplied by the biomedical instrumentation engineer (BMIE), who is on the staff of the kingpin hospital.

The surveillance, guidance, and consultation supplied by a BMIE can be rather costly for individual hospitals to maintain. Recognition of this cost factor and the desire to overcome it has resulted in the development of shared BMIE services.

The kingpin-hospital plan, simply stated, provides for one centrally located hospital (hence "kingpin hospital") to agree to bear the burden of cost and responsibility for placing a BMIE on its staff and sharing his services with member hospitals.

Each member hospital agrees to set up SMI laboratories under the guidance of an engineer and, with his assistance in interviewing and training, hire its own biomedical equipment technicians (BMET's) to operate the laboratory. The fee charged by the kingpin hospital to the member hospitals is just enough to help cover the engineer's salary and partially defray the costs of the SMI capability of the kingpin hospital.

The central-stable concept is very much like that of a commercial, profit-oriented service organization, with the specific exception that it is labeled a nonprofit corporation. This central laboratory is usually well equipped with test instrumentation, mobile equipment, technicians, and clerical and secretarial personnel. Its fees are determined by overhead, salaries, malpractice and negligence insurance premiums, and the cost of handling, stocking, and purchasing replacement parts as well as technician travel to and from member hospitals.

The Goal for Hospitals

All hospitals, regardless of size, should be in a position to certify that any and all instrumentation owned or used by anyone within the hospital is in no way unsafe or hazardous as a result of negligence or carelessness. The aim, regardless of whatever mode is used to accomplish it, should be to provide qualified preventive maintenance, repair, and calibration of all instrumentation.

A true preventive-maintenance program must include a system of data retrieval, periodic recall (retesting), and a means of identifying and locating the equipment covered by the program. The preventive-maintenance system should determine whether all instrumentation covered by it is safe, can be modified to be made safe, or is altogether unsuitable for hospital use, and must therefore be prevented from being used in a hospital.

Regardless of which of the four actual approaches—(1) call system, (2) contract maintenance, (3) shared services, or (4) straight in-house—is used to reach these goals, we must never lose sight of what the hospital administration desires to accomplish. Briefly reiterated, the goal is a program resulting in effective preventive maintenance, repair, calibration, and assurance of utmost safety in the use of all instrumentation.

As an illustration, one might very well ask, "How can one accomplish these aims with a vendor call system service?" It can be done by intensive surveillance of any work performed by the serviceman called in, as well as by requiring documentation indicating symptoms, problems, corrective action, and assurance of calibration. It could possibly follow that the cost of surveillance added to the "future care" cost might very well exceed the expenses incurred by an in-house SMI capability.

How to Get Started

Once it is realized that the goals set down are necessary, then it follows logically to ask how to start to implement a program that will accomplish what is needed.

In the case of the small or medium-sized hospital, depending upon its geographic location (urban, suburban, or rural), the approach might be to look for an existing shared-services program of either a central-stable or kingpin-hospital format in order to initiate an SMI capability; one possible approach is for the hospital to contact its own State Hospital Association or the American Hospital Association for information on BMIE services or plans.

Many seminars and tutorials are given regularly concerning this subject by organizations such as the Association for Advancement of Medical Instrumentation (AAMI), the American Hospital Association (AHA), Bioservice, the Emergency Care Research Institute (ECRI), and state groups such as the Hospital Association of New York State (HANYS) which can provide a suitable background for hospital personnel. Several consultants have become widely known in the field of scientific and medical instrumentation whose aid may be enlisted in setting up a facility in the hospital.

In the case of large hospitals and medical centers, we can recommend two alternate approaches. These are the establishment of a shared-services plan or the establishment of a position on the staff for a BMIE. It is conceivable that by taking into account the number of smaller hospitals within a 75-mile radius of the institution, it might be desirable to have the large medical center take on the role of the kingpin hospital in a shared-services plan.

Maintenance Contracts

The requirement for a maintenance service, both for an instrumentation facility (scientific and medical) as well as for a plant facility has been thoroughly established. Even the smallest nursing home requires at least a handyman or porter to change light bulbs, clean fixtures, replace line-cord plugs, and perform similar typical maintenance functions. An extension of this concept alone to larger institutions provides an indication of the number of skilled and semiskilled personnel needed.

Some maintenance organizations will contract with institutions to perform such maintenance functions. Some of these organizations merely supply supervisory personnel to direct the activities of the hospital's own maintenance personnel. Others offer to perform certain maintenance tasks at regular intervals on a contractual basis. Still other companies offer to perform maintenance and repair work only when called. It is the authors' belief that in theory this type of service appears to be economical and advantageous, and may even be so at the start. However, statistically we have found that it leaves much to be desired. Unless suitable in-house management is available to monitor the activities of an outside maintenance organization, costs will skyrocket, downtime of equipment will increase, meaningful documentation will be lacking, and the overall maintenance program will become unsatisfactory.

An apparent advantage of contract maintenance service is the ability to provide 24-hour service; added advantages are a large centrally located inventory of replacement parts and a guarantee of reduced downtime of equipment. This type of service appears, on the surface, to be lower in actual cost than an in-house capability, but one must give careful consideration to the economics involved.

As noted earlier, a contract service organization must charge enough to cover not only the cost of maintenance but also overhead and profit. The organization must pay its workers' salaries and travel expenses, rental for shop and office space, accountants, malpractice insurance, and utilities, and must, last but not least, show a profit for its owners, providing both compensation and additional money for reinvestment and/or expansion. These funds can come only from the customers who subscribe to the contract service organization.

Actual experience with this type of service has shown many deficiencies. For example, take the case of the hospital that purchased two new sterilizers and also a contract for preventive maintenance and repair. The contract was renewed twice, but at the start of the second renewal a newly appointed director of engineering of the institution made a cost–effectiveness evaluation of the contract.

His investigation revealed that in the preceding 2-year period there were long periods during which the sterilizers had been inoperative, necessitating repeated service calls; that there was a degradation of the machine condition (such as corrosion of solenoid lever bushings, failure of motor mounts and valve packings, timer inaccuracy, etc.) and an overall outward appearance of neglect. The cost for each contract was $2400 per year, plus additional billings for replacement of certain parts. There was one period of downtime that lasted almost two weeks, attributed to a "hard to get" timer. The engineering director questioned the poor condition and appearance of the equipment as well as the justification for the extended out-of-service periods. After several meetings with executives of the service company, both machines, at no additional cost, were overhauled and painted; corroded parts were replaced, leaks were repaired, and the sterilizers began to operate satisfactorily. All this was met with mixed emotions of surprise and joy expressed by the head of the central sterile supply department.

A similar story can be told concerning a service contract for "preventive maintenance" inspections on anesthesia machines. Lack of documentation as supporting evidence of scheduled inspections and inspection procedures, unsatisfactory repairs, and poor overall condition of the machines resulted in cancellation of the service contract. This function was then taken over by in-house BMET's.

These examples, and many others that we could give from our experience, indicates that a qualified individual must be maintained on the hospital staff to monitor closely any and all service agreements by outside organizations in order to obtain effective service. This logically suggests extension of this concept by placing that individual in charge of an in-house or shared-service capability.

When awarding service contracts to outside organizations, the possibility of long delays in providing service also arises because of the need to travel to the hospital requiring such service. The excuse given, for example, for a nine-hour delay in supplying an elevator repairman to one hospital was the energy crisis and difficulty in obtaining gasoline. The organization's service manager, when reprimanded by the chief engineer of the hospital, suggested that they might have in-house electricians perform minor service functions.

Last, but not least, one must be careful of the maintenance contract that covers certain inspections at a fixed fee and merely implies complete coverage. In reality many contracts of this type charge individually for each service call and for parts, so that inspection is not really necessary.

A suitable contract should specify the following:

1. Periodic preventive-maintenance inspections using check lists, with documentation of results and corrective action taken.

2. No additional cost for service calls during weekends, holidays, or off hours.

3. A charge only for parts that have been deliberately broken or rendered inoperative through carelessness of hospital personnel.

4. A guarantee to supply service within a set period of time.

5. Where applicable, a guarantee to supply a "loaner" if repairs require removal of equipment from hospital.

To use a rule of thumb for cost evaluation, the price of the contract annually should not exceed one-eighth the original cost of the equipment. A staff member must be capable of monitoring inspections and service calls.

Shared Services

Shared services, whether a centrally located, nonprofit organization or a kingpin-hospital plan, must by their very nature operate at a lower cost than contract maintenance services.

In the central-stable plan, administrators or associate administrators of the member hospitals are appointed to the board of directors of the shared-service organization, thereby providing a control over fees and parts costs. A modified central-stable plan may even assign service technicians full time to some hospitals, giving them the equivalent of an in-house capability.

The kingpin-hospital program advocates an in-house capability that is carefully guided and monitored from the central hospital. This eliminates travel time for all but the cognizant engineer, who is available for consultation via telephone and in person. The need for transporting equipment from the hospital to a central area and back is eliminated.

The aim of this type of program in a hospital is to establish a scientific and medical instrumentation (SMI) capability.

First, let us define SMI capability as the capacity to:

1. Repair laboratory, medical, and clinical instrumentation.

2. Carry out an effective "preventive maintenance" (PM) program, including data retrieval and proper documentation.

3. Properly and satisfactorily calibrate and/or standardize instrumentation.

4. Perform the foregoing under adverse conditions, e.g., in operating rooms, emergency rooms, etc., as required.

5. Provide for surveillance and guidance by a qualified BMIE.

The foregoing requires that an SMI laboratory be set up in each member hospital and staffed with BMET's. A job description for a BMET will be found in Appendix J.

Figure 7-1 is the layout of a typical SMI laboratory. Uniformity of layout and test equipment is advisable, since it facilitates member hospitals' borrowing technicians when necessary.

The following equipment is the minimum required for hospitals of 100–250 beds and may be expanded for larger hospitals:

1. An EKG signal simulator, approximate price $85.00.

2. A laboratory bench with top shelf, wiremold, and a Masonite top, approximately $210.00.

3. An electronic thermometer (-40 to $302°F$ in three ranges), approximate price $165.00, and an associated probe, approximate price $15.00.

4. A solid-state, battery- and line-operated portable digital voltohmeter (DVOM), approximately $795.00.

5. A stroboscopic tachometer, from 110 to 25,000 rpm, approximate price $310.00.

6. A capacitor substitution box, $25.00; a resistor substitution box, $25.00; and a sine-, triangular-, and square-wave function generator, approximate price $245.00.

7. A voltohmeter, approximately $85.00; a transistor checker attachment for the voltohmeter, approximate cost, $44.00.

8. An electronic tube tester, at an approximate cost of $625.00.

9. A storage oscilloscope, at an approximate cost of $1,370, with a plug-in time-base unit, approximate cost $175; an associated dual-trace plug-in unit, approximate cost $165, and a plug-in differential amplifier, approximate cost $165.00. This is one of the most important items in the SMI laboratory. The storage oscilloscope is used along with sampling circuitry to measure the output of defibrillators, to examine the waveshape and output voltage level of electrosurgical equipment, to check pacemaker waveshape and amplitude, to trouble-shoot electronic monitors and other control equipment, and to conduct preventive-maintenance inspections.

10. An electrical-outlet contact-tension tester selling for approximately $12.50, needed for checking the tension force of outlets throughout the hospital.

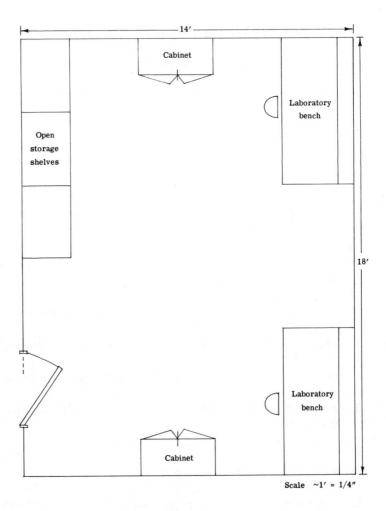

Fig. 7-1   Typical SMI laboratory.

The foregoing items, as stated earlier, make up the basic instrumentation required for a suitable SMI laboratory. There are several lesser items, which are not considered test equipment, but include tools that are necessary for making repairs to instruments. Some of these are the following:

1.   A heavy-duty 4-inch swivel-base vise, approximately $16.00.
2.   A $\frac{3}{8}$-inch electric drill, variable speed, approximately $30.00.
3.   A 6-inch bench grinder, approximately $33.00.

4. A solder gun, approximately $10.00, plus replacement tips.

5. A small soldering-iron handle, with an associated heating unit and several tiplets, approximately $10.00–12.00.

6. A soldering-iron holder at about $2.00.

7. Several types of pliers and two sets of open-end wrenches.

8. Diagonal cutters.

9. Needlenose pliers.

10. Flat-nose pliers.

11. A precision screwdriver kit.

12. A jeweler's screwdriver kit.

13. An automatic center punch.

14. Three 16-drawer cabinets in which to keep small parts (plastic drawer type), about $6.00 each.

Switching over from contract to shared-services maintenance presents no problem. The contracts are either allowed to run out, if they are on an annual basis, or are canceled, if they are self-renewing. This action is instituted gradually as the in-house technicians are prepared to take over the servicing of the equipment.

One means of ensuring that an in-house BMET will later be able to service a particular type of equipment that is covered by contract maintenance is to have the technician present to observe any repairs or maintenance checks made by the contract organization's serviceman. It is even better to have a BMET attend a maintenance training course sponsored by the manufacturer, and many manufacturers provide such training courses. In fact, when purchasing new equipment, it is good practice to insist that the manufacturer provide such training courses at least initially, and preferably on a regular basis. It is also extremely important that the SMI laboratory of any hospital build a complete and comprehensive library of service manuals for all equipment and instrumentation used at the hospital.

Figures 7-2–7-6 show typical setups in an SMI laboratory.

Once a hospital joins a shared-services plan, whether it be of the central-clinical-engineering type or the kingpin plan, it automatically joins in an information pool capable of supplying technical data to the technicians who will perform maintenance checks and repairs for that hospital.

A typical organization chart for a shared-services SMI capability in a member hospital is illustrated in Fig. 7-7.

An integral function of a true shared-services program is the follow-up phase, which involves frequent audits of the SMI capability.

Some advantages of periodic surveys of the SMI laboratory by the

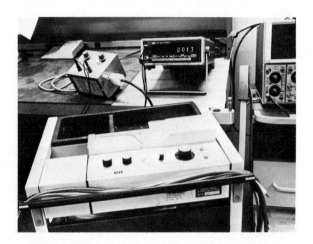

Fig. 7-2   This photograph taken in an SMI laboratory shows a leakage tester attached to an electrocardiograph recorder reading the leakage voltage across a known value of resistance in millivolts on an accurate digital voltmeter.

BMIE are:

1.   Monthly status reports, submitted to the chief engineer, on progress made in maintaining an effective preventive-maintenance program.

2.   Technical advice supplied to SMI technicians for repair of equipment, hazards, etc.

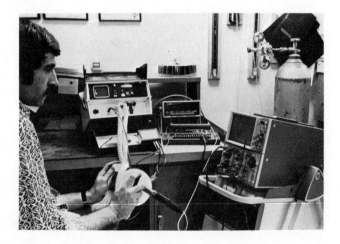

Fig. 7-3   Biomedical equipment technician performing a preventive maintenance check on a portable defibrillator to ascertain whether its output is satisfactory.

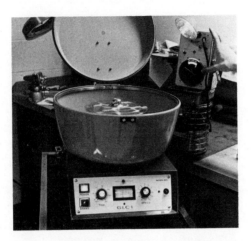

Fig. 7-4 A stroboscope is used to check the performance and speed of a laboratory centrifuge.

3. Data supplied on purchasing instrumentation with respect to optimum economy, safety, and performance.

To get some idea of costs, consider the annual contract for maintenance on operating-room tables and lights for one hospital, which came to $2200. This same service is now performed by a BMET, who is guided by a

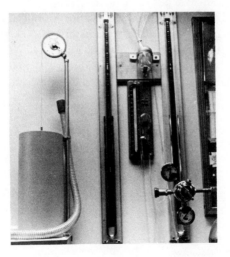

Fig. 7-5 Simple mercury and water manometers are used for the measurement of pressure. Note spirometer to the left for measurement of gas volumes.

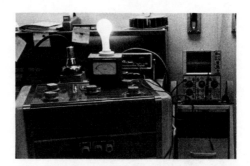

Fig. 7-6 A load lamp, radio-frequency current meter, and oscilloscope are utilized in the performance test of an electrosurgical apparatus.

shared-services BMIE at an approximate labor cost of only $250 annually or 89% less than the contract maintenance cost.

When one considers the cost of a maintenance contract for an individual type of equipment wherein preventive maintenance and repairs will be performed, one can assume a minimum cost of a typical agreement to be somewhere in the range of $1200 to $2400 annually. The average community hospital having 200–300 beds, covering both medical and laboratory instrumentation, would have to carry anywhere from 10 to 20 maintenance contracts. By extrapolation, this would indicate an annual overall fee in the range of $24,000 to $48,000. Then, too, one must consider that this would only cover 10–20 types of instrumentation.

In the light of this analysis, let us assume an initial cost of setting up a minimal SMI laboratory at approximately $6,000 and the salary for two technicians at approximately $20,000 annually. We can then logically assign an initial start-up cost of $26,000 for the first year for an SMI capability. It should, however, be noted that this only covers not the

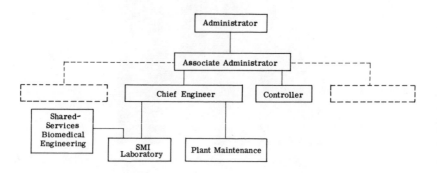

Fig. 7-7 Organization chart for a shared-services SMI capability.

10–20 types of instrumentation used for the comparison, but will eventually cover all instrumentation in the hospital that is within the jurisdiction of the preventive-maintenance program.

Comparison of the cost of shared-services versus that of contract maintenance for biomedical instrumentation reveals that the very structure of the latter form of service results in higher costs as previously shown with plant maintenance.

Of inestimable value in a shared-services plan is the engineering advice available for the purchase of new instrumentation and hospital equipment. The shared-services instrumentation engineer sincerely desires that there be a minimum of repairs and a maximum of preventive maintenance on equipment. His frequent visits to the member hospitals involving consultation and problem-solving for a myriad of instrument difficulties makes him well-qualified to evaluate performance, serviceability, and overall engineering design. An illustrative example of how valuable this capability can be is the story of a member hospital that was about to purchase a specific fetal monitoring system because their chief of obstetrics felt this type was the best. The shared-services engineer advised against that particular model and manufacturer because he was aware of continuous and repeated problems with this very same system in another member hospital. He had even noted specific design deficiencies in the recording system. Systems of this type have practically no resale value, so that it behooves the buyer to make a wise choice and assure himself of the greatest trouble-free utilization when purchasing such equipment.

In-House Maintenance

In-house maintenance means that personnel required to perform preventive maintenance repairs and calibration of equipment are employed by the institution on a full-time basis. The only difference between this and the kingpin-hospital shared-services program is that instead of a biomedical engineer monitoring and guiding the program on a shared basis, such an engineer is employed on a full time basis by the hospital.

The additional salary of the engineer could range anywhere from $18,000 to $25,000 per year. Therefore, complete in-house capability is usually found only in the kingpin hospital of a shared-engineering-services plan or in a large medical center.

The advantages of an in-house maintenance capability are identical to those of shared engineering services that require the hospital to establish their own SMI laboratory manned by BMET's. The technicians in the in-house laboratory come under the jurisdiction of a biomedical engineer, who is usually responsible to the administration only.

To compare the savings in negligence suits versus the cost of an SMI capability, consider the hospital whose electrician installed a new line cord and plug on a therapeutic muscle stimulator. It supplies pulses of electricity to conductive wet sponges affixed to the body in the region of the muscle to be activated. The pulse width and repetition rate are adjustable, and the amplitude of the pulse is variable up to approximately 30 V. However, this pulse is derived from a differential voltage between two grid-controlled vacuum tubes whose plates are at 280 V dc with respect to circuit ground, which is connected to an internal, isolated chassis.

The line cord (which originally was 2-wire) enters this chassis through an insulated strain-relief bushing. The chassis is completely enclosed by, but insulated from, a sloped-front cabinet with controls mounted on the sloped panel.

The electrician, not understanding the circuitry involved, grounded the isolated chassis via the 3-wire cord and 3-prong plug. This converted the machine to a potentially lethal device capable of shocking a patient with 280 V dc from a well-regulated power supply if he were to contact ground.

An accident of this type could be proven to be sheer negligence resulting from incompetence. BMET's have grounded the outer case of these machines without grounding the inner chassis. Their care in doing so evolves from engineering guidance as well as the ability to comprehend circuit schematics and electronic circuitry.

The SMI laboratory of a typical 250-bed community hospital should have a minimum of two in-house BMET's, as was previously indicated in the section dealing with hospital size.

Discussion of in-house maintenance for any health-care facility must and should encompass building maintenance. The need for on-the-spot repairs and preventive-maintenance inspections of all plant equipment is obvious. Renovations and modifications to various areas of the hospital could involve plumbing, electrical, and carpentry skills, which are usually supplied by the maintenance engineering department.

Contract plant maintenance, if it could be obtained, would in all likelihood be prohibitive in cost and in almost all cases found to be impractical. The result is that practically every hospital has a maintenance engineering department.

Obvious advantages attributable to this type of operation are not limited to money savings but also encompass possibly even more valuable time savings. Of course this holds true only if the maintenance engineering department is properly managed and works toward realistic goals.

The building maintenance department, or maintenance engineering, is closely related to patient, personnel, and visitor safety. Inefficiency or incompetence in its operation can readily lead to unsafe and, in some cases, hazardous situations.

For example, envisage an improperly scheduled assignment of maintenance personnel in response to repair requests. The men do not have time to complete or properly handle emergency repairs, and this situation creates an atmosphere conducive to accidents. For example, a broken step edge remains unrepaired until a nurse suffers a serious fall. An examination lamp is supposed to be modified to a 3-wire grounded system, but the conversion is postponed and nearly causes an electrocution. Or how about the maintenance electrician who does not have time to properly replace a ground wire to a bed outlet in the ICU. The patient in the bed connected to that outlet has a catheter in his heart!

Well then, how do we start to make a maintenance engineering department efficient? The following basic concepts must be implemented if they do not already exist.

1. A service or job requisition slip, properly filled in, must be submitted to the maintenance engineering (ME) dispatcher. The dispatcher, who also serves as a parts clerk, is responsible for the parts-and-materials stockroom, answers phone calls, logs in service requisitions, and dispatches maintenance mechanics to various jobs.

2. All service requisitions must be assigned job numbers and logged in. A sample maintenance work-order log is shown in Fig. 7-8. An estimated completion time and a priority are given to each job by the dispatcher.

3. The priority system adopted by some efficient groups uses the letters A, B, C, and D. A indicates an immediate priority. B stands for completion within 24 hours. C requires completion within one week. D requires scheduling by the chief engineer, e.g., renovations and alterations.

4. Where possible, a maintenance man should be on duty for the 4-to-midnight shift to handle minor emergencies such as stopped-up toilets, plumbing leaks, blown fuses, visitors locked in elevators, circuit breakers that have kicked out, etc.

5. Between the hours of midnight and 8 a.m. it is advisable to have a maintenance mechanic on call for problems similar to those in (4) above.

At Nyack Hospital, a telephone-answering set has been installed in the ME dispatcher's office, adjacent to that of the Chief Engineer. This unit employs a separate announcement tape, which, after the first ring, states:

"This is the Maintenance Engineering Office. If your message is of utmost urgency, such as flooding, imminent danger, etc., please call the operator.

If it is not that urgent, then at the sound of the tone, please state the time, your name, the nature and location of the problem, and your extension. The matter will be given attention first thing in the morning. Thank you."

A second tape, on a cassette, records the message or complaint. The cassette is played back the following morning, and priorities are assigned to problems received.

Now all of this deals with the immediate task of improving efficiency and handling repairs and breakdowns as they occur, but this is not the long-range approach to the overall proplem. The system that reduces the number of breakdowns, increases the mean time between failures (MTBF), and improves the safety factor is *preventive maintenance* (PM). This term is used by many service organizations that do not actually supply true preventive maintenance. True PM cannot exist without honest inspections performed at set frequencies and accompanied by meaningful documentation.

If one were to check with the SMI departments of such hospitals as Downstate Medical Center, Brooklyn, New York; Phelps Memorial Hospital, North Tarrytown, New York; Nyack Hospital, Nyack, New York; and others that have initiated PM programs, the information obtained would statistically prove that preventive maintenance of complex instrumentation has reduced the number of repairs and breakdowns. At Nyack Hospital we therefore extended the approach to plant maintenance.

Each and every pump, motor, fan, blower, air conditioner, cart, heater,

Maintenance Work Order Log

W. C. No.	Request By	Date Rec'd.	Date Req'd.	Description	Act. Hrs.	Prior.	Men Assigned	Est. M/H	Date Start	Comp

Fig. 7-8 Maintenance work-order log.

alarm system, etc. is tagged with an ME tag. This is a Metalcal label on which is typed a maintenance-engineering number. For each ME number, a preventive-maintenance card is filled out with item name, description, manufacturer, model number, and location. Numerical coding is assigned to item name or category, manufacturer, and location. Frequency of inspection is also assigned and punched into the Keysort card. See Fig. 7-9 which illustrates the Metalcal tag and the card.

This system is compatible for use with a digital computer for indicating which equipment is due for inspection—monthly, quarterly, or annually. However, even if no computer is available, the Keysort card provides a rapid means of performing this function as well as providing statistical data. Without data retrieval, there is no way to determine the effectiveness and cost savings of a preventive-maintenance program.

Present-Day Maintenance Organizations

Safety, maintenance, and repair in the modern hospital are not limited to scientific and medical instrumentation alone. The building-maintenance department carries a large share of the responsibility for safety in the hospital.

We have advocated and maintain that it is important to keep the two functions—SMI laboratory and maintenance enginering department—distinct and separate. The complexity and sophistication of the former versus the semiskilled requirements of the latter mean that only an individual capable of exercising excellent judgment as well as technical understanding can successfully manage both groups.

A very recent trend appearing in several large hospitals is to appoint a Director of Engineering Services. Ideally this individual should have an extensive background in scientific and medical instrumentation theory and a good foundation in the physical sciences. Figure 7-10 indicates the location of this position in a typical organizational chart. The extent of responsibility given to the Director of Engineering Services is naturally dependent upon the hospital's size. It is a recognizable fact that the modern hospital must tighten up on security in light of the drug situation and the rash of losses of all types as a result of thefts. The Director of Engineering Services may be in a position to contribute substantially to the enhancement of security if he has the requisite ingenuity and engineering background to determine the type of monitoring and alarm systems required. The BMI laboratory should obviously be his responsibility, on the basis of his BMI engineering background and his ability to fully comprehend the

Hospital Preventive Maintenance Card - Maintenance Engineering Dept.

	M. E. No.				
1. Equipment Name	Cat. No.				
2. Manufacturer	Manufacturers Code No.				

3. Description

4. Type or Model No.		Serial No.	

5. Location	Location No.		Fixed Portable

6. Preventive Maintenance Schedule

   6.1) Minor   6.1.1) Monthly ☐   6.1.2) Quarterly ☐   6.1.3) Semi-annual ☐

   6.2) Major   6.2.1) Quarterly ☐   6.2.2) Semi-annual ☐   6.2.3) Annual ☐

7. Maintenance Procedure Required   7.1) Minor (Form No.) _____

                                          7.2) Major (Form No.) _____

8. Date of Last Inspection (Month, Day, Year)

9. Failure Record

   9.1) Last Failure Date (Month, Day, Year)

   9.2) Component Failure   Date

NYACK HOSPITAL
Engineering Services Department
ME No. [9156]

Fig. 7-9a Hospital preventive-maintenance card (front side) and equipment tag.

basic principles of this type of instrumentation as well as his awareness of possible hazards that may exist with the equipment. The Chief Engineer or Director of Maintenance should definitely report to the Director of Engineering Services, since the maintenance activity in a hospital is closely interlinked with safety and repair of equipment and can benefit from liaison with the aforementioned activities. As indicated by the chart, the Director of Engineering Services is responsible only to Administration.

When this type of organizational order exists in a hospital surrounded (approximately in a 50- to 75-mile radius) by small or medium-sized hospitals, then a shared BMI engineering program could very well come

9.3) Performance Failures (Reasons Other Than 9.2)	Date

10. Repair Costs

10.1) Cost of Material   10.2) Main Hours

(a) _____ (f) _____ (k) _____ (p) _____   (a) _____ (f) _____ (k) _____ (p) _____

(b) _____ (g) _____ (l) _____ (q) _____   (b) _____ (g) _____ (l) _____ (q) _____

(c) _____ (h) _____ (m) _____ (r) _____   (c) _____ (h) _____ (m) _____ (r) _____

(d) _____ (i) _____ (n) _____ (s) _____   (d) _____ (i) _____ (n) _____ (s) _____

(e) _____ (j) _____ (o) _____ (t) _____   (e) _____ (j) _____ (o) _____ (t) _____

11. Preventive Main Cost of Materials

(a) _____ (e) _____ (i) _____ (m) _____ (q) _____ (u) _____

(b) _____ (f) _____ (j) _____ (n) _____ (r) _____ (v) _____

(c) _____ (g) _____ (k) _____ (o) _____ (s) _____ (w) _____

(d) _____ (h) _____ (l) _____ (p) _____ (t) _____ (x) _____

COMMENTS:

Fig. 7-9b   Hospital preventive-maintenance card (reverse side).

under the direction of the individual who is the Director of Engineering Services for a central hospital. Figure 7-11 is the organizational chart for the Engineering Services section of Nyack Hospital, Nyack, New York, and clearly illustrates the order of responsibility in a hospital of just under 400 beds.

If we examine the detailed duties and responsibilities of the key personnel in the organizational arrangement depicted in Fig. 7-11 we find the Chief Engineer responsible for:

1.   Building wiring in accord with the National Electrical Code and specific bulletins of the NFPA relating to hospitals.

2.   Proper operation and maintenance of boilers.

3.   Maintenance and checking of a satisfactory emergency power-generating system.

4.   Operation and maintenance of heating, ventilating, and air-conditioning equipment.

5.   Maintenance and appearance of grounds.

6.   Painting and decorating of all areas of the hospital.

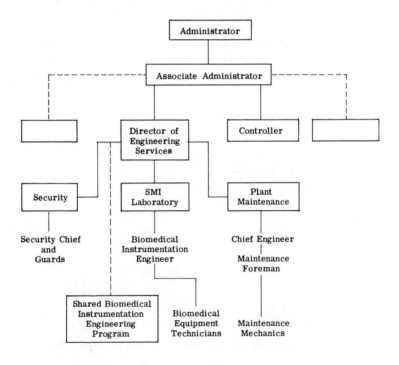

Fig. 7-10   Typical organization chart.

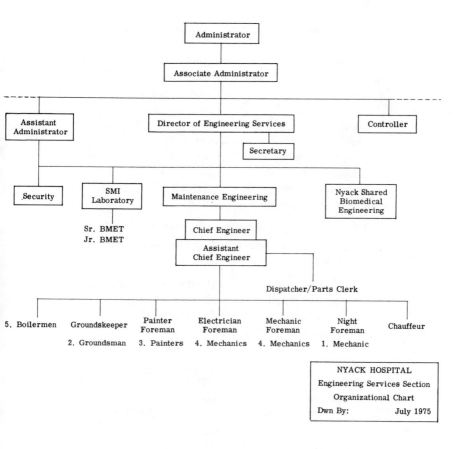

Fig. 7-11 Organization chart for Nyack Hospital.

7. Maintenance, repair, and safe operation of all stretchers, wheel chairs, etc.

(Note: All of the foregoing are directly or indirectly involved in maintaining safety in the hospital.)

The BMET is responsible for:

1. Carrying out a preventive-maintenance program as delineated by and under the guidance of a BMIE, who might be the Director of Engineering Services or supplied by a shared-services program from a neighboring hospital. This program involves complex testing and calibration of sophisticated biomedical instrumentation.

2.   Repairing or modifying equipment and instruments, both electrical and mechanical, to ensure safety.

3.   Maintaining a uniform record system of preventive maintenance and repairs as well as work-progress logs.

4.   Performing initial check-outs of new equipment purchased by the hospital.

5.   Instructing doctors, nurses, and other medical personnel in the proper and safe use and care of instrumentation as outlined by the BMIE.

6.   Assisting physicians in setting up and operating specialized electronic equipment.

7.   Working on instrumentation in the OR, ICU, or CCU under emergency or adverse conditions.

The need for security guards dictates for either a Sergeant, Lieutenant, or Captain of the Guards, dependent upon hospital size and location, to be responsible for:

1.   Keeping unauthorized personnel from entering areas where their safety or the safety of patients is affected.

2.   Checking operation of elevators after regular hours and calling service organization when required.

3.   Preventing theft of drugs, instrumentation, and office equipment from the hospital.

4.   Directing traffic near the emergency entrance to ensure speedy discharge of patients from ambulances.

5.   Restraining disturbed patients, who sometimes injure nursing personnel or fellow patients.

The Director of Engineering Services, through the departments reporting to him, is responsible for:

1.   A scientific and medical instrumentation capability involving patient and personnel safety.

2.   An efficiently operating maintenance organization geared to rapid repair and a preventive-maintenance program for plant equipment and instruments leading to a safe hospital.

3.   Security operations intended to reduce or eliminate accidents, thefts, fire hazards, and even bomb threats.

4.   Reviewing specifications, bids, drawings, etc. for additions, renovations or major alterations with respect to electrical, mechanical, and fire safety.

One might very well question the need for the Director of Engineering Services to review the specifications and drawings supplied to the hospital by registered, licensed architects and engineers. That such a need exists is best demonstrated by the true story of a hospital that engaged a firm of architects to initiate specifications and blueprints for an electrical contractor to make a modification. The modification was intended to permit operation of "special-procedure" X-ray equipment on emergency power. The contractor completed the job in accord with the prints he was supplied with by the electrical engineers, but the X-ray equipment would not operate on emergency power because the generator could not supply the surges demanded from it and recover before recycling.

How does this relate to safety? Ask the patient lying on the X-ray table with a catheter in his heart when a power failure takes place. This illustration is not meant to imply that architects and engineers are incompetent but rather that even they can make mistakes occasionally. If the infrequent mistake involving safety can be avoided, the hospital benefits.

The Overall Aspect of Safety

We hope that we do not leave the reader believing that safety in health-care institutions is strictly limited to medical instrumentation, electric shock, etc. However, along with these particular hazards, if one were to list all other possible areas for accidents to occur, one would have to add to these areas all of the standard hazards that exist in public buildings per se. It is for this reason alone that the Director of Engineering Services, or any person who has responsibilities similar to his, should play an active role on the safety committee of the institution. An example of some of the contributions this person can make to the safety committee is provided by the story of an accident report being read at a safety-committee meeting indicating that this particular hospital had glass shelves above the sinks in patient bathrooms. A patient placed a bottle on the glass shelf rather vigorously, breaking the glass, which resulted in his foot being cut. The following week a program replacing all the glass shelves with clear lucite shelves was instituted. There is also the situation that existed in one hospital where the inhalation therapy department insisted on storing their oxygen tanks without protective caps on them. The Director of Engineering Services was very insistent upon the protective cap being placed on each tank that was stored; he actually furnished further supporting data for this proposed safety measure, pointing out that the weakest point in the tank is at the valve location, and that explosions have been known to occur when such tanks have fallen over.

We can see that responsibility for safety in the hospital lies with the hospital or health-care institution, and as more and more institutions initiate preventive-maintenance and safety programs, there will be no explanation other than negligence for not providing such programs.

Bibliography

AAMI Tutorial on Biomedical Equipment and Technology at the Statler Hilton Hotel, New York. (Oct. 31–Nov. 2, 1973).

Butler vs. Northwestern Hospital of Minneapolis, 202 MINN. 282 278 N.W. 37.

Developing a Hospital Medical Equipment Maintenance Program, *Med. Instrum.* **7,** No. 1 (Jan.–Feb. 1973).

Fischmann, G. S., What's Wrong with the Biomedical Instrument Market, *Inst. Tech.* **16,** No. 8 (Aug. 1969).

Kane, I. M., Nyack Shared Biomedical Instrumentation Engineering Plan, 26th ACEMB, Minneapolis, Minnesota (Sept. 30, 1973).

Kauffman, H. D., Planned Preventive Maintenance and Electrical Safety Testing, *Med. Electron. Equip. News* **19,** No. 8 (Aug. 1974).

Lubin, D., The Hospital Engineer and Electrical Safety in the Hospital, *Hospital Eng.* **12,** No. 11 (Nov. 1967).

Norton, M. L., Biomedical Instrumentation and Liability, *J. Ass. Advanc. Med. Instrum.* (May–June 1971).

Appendix A

CALIBRATION OF DC AND AC METERS

A dc meter will read the average value of current or voltage. Since dc values do not vary a great deal as a rule about a mean value, i.e., their fluctuation is usually small, the accuracy of a dc-meter reading will be largely a function of the accurate calibration of the meter. A dc meter cannot, however, be used to measure ac directly, since it measures an average value, and the average value of an ac waveform is zero.

The waveform shown in Fig. A-1, a typical ac 60 Hz waveform with a peak value of 155.58 V, must be rectified prior to measurement by a meter; the full-wave rectified ac waveform is shown in Fig. A-2. It will be seen that rectification merely inverts the negative-going part of the waveform. Since the same type of meter is still used to measure the voltage or current, it will show the *average* voltage or current, which in this case (voltage being illustrated), is 99.25 V. In ac measurements we are interested, however, to obtain the root mean square (rms) value of the voltage. As has already been stated, the rms value of a sine-wave voltage is 0.707 its peak value, or $0.707 \times 155.58 = 110$ V. In order for the dc meter, which reads the average value of the rectified ac voltage, to indicate an rms voltage instead, the meter must be recalibrated so that an *actual* voltage of 99.25 V, the true *average* voltage of the rectified waveform shown in Fig. A-2, is *indicated* as 110 V. The meter will be seen to be calibrated higher by the ratio of 110/99.25, or roughly by a factor of 1.11. This is, of course, exactly what was wanted, but if this recalibrated meter is now used to measure dc values, it will read these d.c. values erroneously, since its calibration has been purposely altered to provide a higher reading. In an application where one and the same meter is used interchangeably to read either dc or ac values, a voltage divider must be provided ahead of the meter to reduce the actual dc voltage by a factor of 99.25/110, or approximately 0.905. This is shown in Fig. A-3.

153

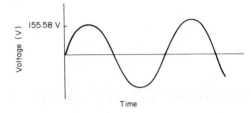

Fig. A-1. Conventional 60-Hz, 110-V rms waveform.

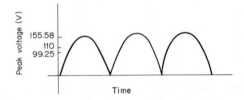

Fig. A-2. Rectified waveform of Fig. A-1.

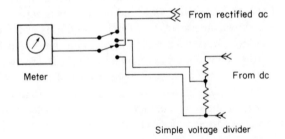

Fig. A-3. Meter used interchangeably as ac or dc meter.

Appendix B

VOLTAGE AND CURRENT RELATIONSHIPS FOR RESISTANCE, CAPACITANCE, AND INDUCTANCE

The relationship between voltage and current for a resistance has already been covered in Chapter 2; i.e. $V/I = R$. This is a linear relationship independent of time; i.e., the ratio of voltage V to current I is true no matter what the magnitude of the voltage is, and it will hold true for any instant of time. If the voltage changes with time, so will the current, and this relationship is considered to be time-independent.

The voltage–current relationship for a capacitance or an inductance is, however, time-dependent, because time enters into the equation. We must therefore introduce the concept of the time derivative, which is simply the rate of change with respect to time. For example, Fig. B-1 shows a voltage changing linearly with respect to time; it increases in, say, 10 sec from 0 to 100 V. What is the rate of change of this voltage? It is the total voltage change—i.e., from 0 to 100 V, or 100 V—divided by the time it took to change from 0 to 100 V—i.e., by 10 sec. The rate of change of voltage is therefore

$$100 \text{ V}/10 \text{ sec} = 10 \text{ V}/\text{sec}$$

The rate of change of voltage happens to be constant for this example at any point along the curve. Thus, if the 2-sec interval is examined where the voltage changed from 60 to 80 V, the rate of change of this voltage will be $(80 - 60)$ V/2 sec, which is again 20 V/2 sec or 10 V/sec.

Hence the difference in voltage V over the difference in time t is the rate of change of voltage with respect to time, or the voltage time derivative. The voltage time derivative for the example shown in Fig. B-1 will be the same, i.e., 10 V/sec, no matter how small the interval chosen on the line. For example, we would obtain the same results if we measured the voltage change from 60 to 61 V over a time interval of 0.1 sec.

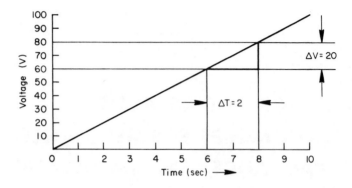

Fig. B-1   Concept of time derivative.

In the limit—i.e., if the interval chosen is very small—we write dV/dt, meaning that this is the time derivative for the voltage at a particular chosen point. Although the point at which we choose the voltage derivative is irrelevant in the case of Fig. B-1, this is not always the case. Figure B-2 shows, for example, a curve that is termed "exponentially rising." Here the voltage derivative will vary, depending on where on that curve the derivative is measured.

A matter of particular interest is the time derivative of a sine wave. This is shown in Fig. B-3.

In order to obtain a better physical understanding of the meaning of the derivative, four points, 1–4, are shown on the sine wave described by the expression $\sin \omega t$, and four corresponding points, labeled 1A–4A, are shown on the derivative of $\sin \omega t$, which is $\omega \cos \omega t$. At this time, it will be seen that

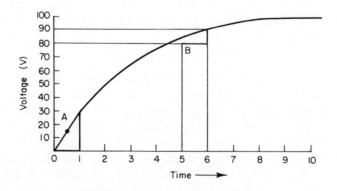

Fig. B-2   Derivative of an exponentially rising waveform. The derivative at point A has a different value than that at point B.

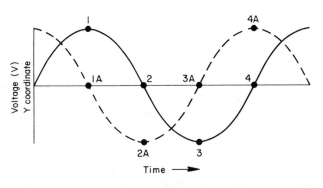

Fig. B-3 Illustration of the derivative of a sine wave. —, sin ωt; – – – , d/dt (sin ωt) = cos ωt.

the sine wave peaks at point 1, and consequently its time derivative is zero (the slope is zero), as can be seen from point 1A, the Y coordinate of which is zero. At point 2 the sine wave shows its greatest negative slope, and the time derivative consequently shows a negative maximum at point 2A. At point 3 the slope of the sine wave is again zero, and the time derivative seen at point 3A is consequently also zero. At point 4 the sine wave exhibits its maximum positive slope, and hence the time derivative at point 4A also exhibits its maximum value. It is of interest to note that the derivative of a sine wave is de facto a displaced sine wave; that sine wave, displaced by 90°, and leading the original sine wave by 90°, is a cosine wave, the equation of which is ω cos ωt. By corollary, the derivative of a cosine wave, i.e.

$$d/dt \ (\cos \omega t) \ = \ -\omega \sin \omega t$$

is an inverted sine wave, or a sine wave with a minus sign in front of it.

We are now ready to examine in more detail the voltage–current relationship existing in resistors, inductors, and capacitors. These can be stated as follows:

$$V = IR$$

denoting that the voltage applied across a resistor is equal to the product of the resistance R and the current I;

$$V = L \, dI/dt$$

denoting that the voltage across an inductor is equal to the product of the value of the inductor L and the time derivative of the current I flowing through the inductor;

$$I = C \, dV/dt$$

denoting that the current flowing through a capacitor is equal to the product of the value of the capacitor C and the time derivative of the voltage V across the capacitor.

With these facts, let us reexamine the examples given in Chapter 2. Given a voltage equal to $V = 100 \sin \omega t$, what is the peak current it will produce when applied across a capacitor equal to 1 μF, or 1×10^{-6} farads?

We know that $I = C\, dV/dt$; substituting actual values into this formula, we obtain

$$I = C\, dV/dt = C\, d/dt\, (100 \sin \omega t) = C\omega\, 100 \cos \omega t = 1 \times 10^{-6}$$

$$\times 377 \cos 377t$$

$$= 0.0377 \cos \omega t \text{ amp} \qquad \text{or} \quad 37.7 \text{ mA}$$

The rms value of that current will be $0.707 \times 0.0377 = 26.6$ mA. This relationship is plotted in Fig. B-4.

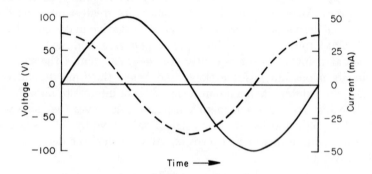

Fig. B-4   The current leads the voltage by 90° when a sine-wave voltage is impressed on a capacitor. Since $I_i = C\, dv/dt$, $I_i = 0.0377 \cos \omega t$ (- - -) when $V = 100 \sin \omega t$ (—).

Appendix C

APPLICATION OF KIRCHHOFF'S LAWS TO THE WHEATSTONE BRIDGE

A wheatstone bridge is commonly used to determine the value of an unknown resistance, for example R_4, if the values of resistances R_1, R_2, and R_3 are known (see Fig. C-1). By placing a current meter in series with resistor R_5 and varying any other calibrated resistor, i.e., either R_1, R_2, or R_3, it is possible to determine the value of the unknown resistor R_4 by adjusting the value of the variable resistor until the current meter shows a zero value of current. At this point it can be shown that $R_1/R_3 = R_2/R_4$, i.e., the voltage at the junction of R_1 and R_3 equals the voltage at the junction of R_2 and R_4 so that there is no potential difference across resistor R_5, and consequently no current can flow in it. How would one work out the current in R_5 if that relationship did not hold—i.e., if R_1/R_3 were not equal to R_2/R_4? This particular example is worked out below, and is a good illustration of the application of Kirchhoff's laws.

The first thing to do is to assume some currents flowing in the network, and it is interesting to note that one need not even be correct about the assumed direction of the current flow: if the assumption is wrong, the current flow will turn out to be negative, showing that it flows in the opposite direction from that originally assumed.

An assumed current flow is shown in Fig. C-2; it will be seen that it is assumed that the current, on leaving resistor R_1, divides its flow in a fashion as yet to be determined between resistors R_3 and R_5; on leaving resistor R_5, that current combines with the current flowing through resistor R_2, the combined current flowing through resistor R_4.

Based on these assumptions, and using Kirchhoff's laws the following three equations will hold:

$$\text{Loop 1} \qquad I_1R_1 + (I_1 - I_3)R_3 - V = 0 \qquad (1)$$

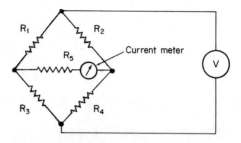
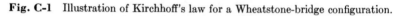

Fig. C-1 Illustration of Kirchhoff's law for a Wheatstone-bridge configuration.

$$\text{Loop 2} \qquad I_2R_2 + (I_2 + I_3)R_4 - V = 0 \qquad\qquad (2)$$

$$\text{Loop 3} \qquad I_1R_1 + I_3R_5 - I_2R_2 \qquad\quad = 0 \qquad\qquad (3)$$

From Eq. (3),

$$I_1 = (I_2R_2 - I_3R_5)/R_1 \qquad\qquad (4)$$

Substituting into Eq. (1), multiplying by R_1, and collecting terms, we get

$$I_2(R_1R_2 + R_2R_3) - I_3(R_1R_5 + R_3R_5 + R_1R_3) - VR_1 = 0 \qquad\qquad (5)$$

From Eq. (2),

$$I_2 = (V - I_3R_4)/(R_2 + R_4) \qquad\qquad (6)$$

Substituting Eq. (6) into Eq. (5), multiplying by $(R_2 + R_4)$, and collecting terms, we obtain

$$V(R_2R_3 - R_1R_4) - I_3(R_1R_2R_4 + R_2R_3R_4 + R_2R_3R_5 + R_1R_4R_5$$
$$+ R_3R_4R_5 + R_1R_3R_4 + R_1R_2R_5 + R_1R_2R_3) = 0 \qquad (7)$$

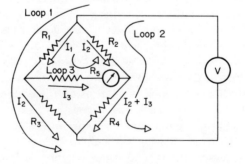

Fig. C-2 Calculation of current flow: assumptions: $I_3 = (I_1 - I_2)$ flowing into R_5; $(I_2 + I_3)$ flowing into R_4.

or

$$I_3 = \frac{V(R_2R_3 - R_1R_4)}{R_1R_2R_4 + R_2R_3R_4 + R_2R_3R_5 + R_1R_4R_5 + R_3R_4R_5 + R_1R_3R_4 + R_1R_2R_5 + R_1R_2R_3} \qquad (8)$$

From Eq. (8) it will be seen that if R_1/R_3 does in fact equal R_2/R_4, then $R_2R_3 = R_1R_4$, the numerator of I_3 will be zero, and I_3 will also be zero. If R_2R_3 is greater than R_1R_4, the current flow of I_3 will be positive, and our original assumption will have been correct. If R_1R_4 is greater than R_2R_3, the current flow of I_3 will be negative, meaning that I_3 really flows from the junction of R_2 and R_4 into the junction of R_1 and R_3.

Assume now that $V = 10\ V$, $R_1 = 1000$ ohms, $R_2 = 2000$ ohms, $R_3 = 3000$ ohms, and $R_5 = 500$ ohms. What will be the value of I_3, the current registered by the current meter?

According to Eq. (8), we get

$$I_3 = \frac{10(6 \times 10^6 - 4 \times 10^6)}{10^9(8 + 24 + 30 + 20 + 60 + 12 + 10 + 6)} = \frac{2 \times 10^7}{168 \times 10^9}$$

$$= 0.119 \times 10^{-3}\ \text{amp}$$

$$= 0.119\ \text{mA}$$

Appendix D

DEFIBRILLATORS AND THEIR WAVEFORMS

Shaping circuits, using transient waveforms, are used by defibrillators in one form or another, usually deriving energy from a charged capacitor. The simplest discharge circuit is a resistance–capacitance (RC) circuit, shown for illustrative purposes only in Fig. D-1.

Figure D-2 illustrates the discharge voltage or current of the circuit of Fig. D-1; this discharge current dies away gradually when switch S is closed, the discharge current flowing through resistor R. The type of gradual current or voltage decay shown in Fig. D-2 is also referred to as exponential decay.

The earliest type of defibrillator used the discharge circuit shown in Fig. D-1; because of the very high initial voltage compared to the available energy in the discharge pulse, this type of defibrillator is no longer in use today. The energy in the discharge pulse is given by

$$\text{energy} = W = \tfrac{1}{2}CV^2 = 500 \text{ watt-sec or joules}$$

for $V = 5000$ V and C $= 40$ μF.

The 50-ohm load resistor R_L simulates the resistance of the human body.

The most widely used defibrillator circuit is the so-called RLC defibrillator (resistance, inductance, and capacitance). In its simplest form it consists of a dc power supply, a storage capacitor, a series inductor (inclusive of its resistance), and a load resistor. This circuit is shown in Fig. D-3, its discharge waveform in Fig. D-4.

The energy contained in this circuit is again given by

$$\text{energy} = W = \tfrac{1}{2}CV^2 = 500 \text{ W-sec}$$

for a charging voltage of 5000 V and a capacitor value of 40 μF. Because the inductor L has resistance and is therefore lossy, the amount of energy delivered to the patient, who is assumed to have a resistance of 50 ohms,

162

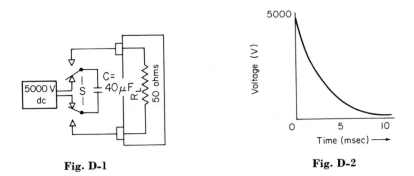

Fig. D-1

Fig. D-2

Fig. D-1 Simple RC discharge circuit.
Fig. D-2 Discharge waveform for circuit of Fig. D-1.

is 250 W-sec at a maximum discharge voltage of 1840 V for the values given, i.e. a voltage considerably less than the charging voltage of the capacitor.

By modifying the values of R, L, and C it is possible to modify the waveform to the "underdamped" form shown in Fig. D-5, a waveform frequently used in defibrillators.

Another type of defibrillator waveform is derived by means of a delay line. The circuit for a delay-line defibrillator is shown in Fig. D-6, its waveform in Fig. D-7. The effect of the double L–C combination is to increase the rise and fall time of the waveform and also to broaden it out, thus delivering more energy at a lower peak voltage.

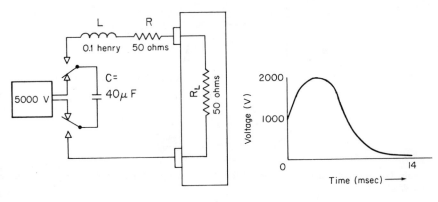

Fig. D-3

Fig. D-4

Fig. D-3 RLC defibrillator.
Fig. D-4 Discharge waveform of RLC defibrillator.

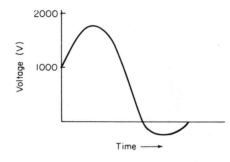

Fig. D-5 Discharge waveform of underdamped RLC defibrillator.

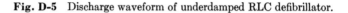

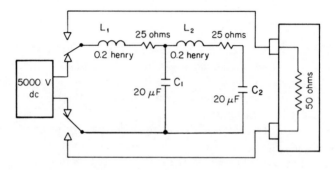

Fig. D-6 Delay-line defibrillator.

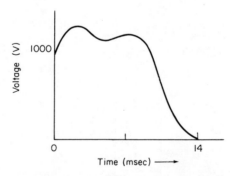

Fig. D-7 Waveform of delay-line defibrillator. Energy stored $= \frac{1}{2}(C_1 + C_2)V^2 =$ 500 W-sec.

Appendix E

REMOTE TRANSMISSION OF HEARTBEATS BY TELEMETRY

A typical heartbeat waveform is shown in Fig. E-1. This waveform cannot, however, be transmitted directly to a receiver for the simple reason that a frequency of 70 Hz or so, which is a typical frequency of a heartbeat, does not propagate over the air easily. It is possible, however, to transmit considerably higher frequencies over the air; by modulating such a high-frequency carrier with the intelligence—in this case EKG information from a patient—it is possible to transmit the intelligence. One of the bands allotted for transmission of industrial, scientific, and medical information by the Federal Communications Commission (FCC) is the 174–216 MHz band, and the majority of medical telemetry equipment makes use of this band. An unmodulated carrier is shown in Fig. E-2; the same carrier modulated by a typical heartbeat waveform is shown in Fig. E-3.

A typical telemetry system for the transmission of heartbeats from patients is shown in Fig. E-4. The sensor in this case consists of electrodes, picking up the information from the patient; the difference potential between two electrodes is typically a waveform depicted in Fig. E-1. This waveform is then amplified by an amplifier, preferably a difference amplifier, and fed to the modulator. The modulator has another input fed to it from a carrier-frequency generator, usually an oscillator oscillating at the carrier frequency, normally at an FCC approved frequency in the 174–216 MHz region. The oscillator output represents the unmodulated carrier, as shown in Fig. E-2. It is the function of the modulator to modulate the carrier in accordance with the information coming from the sensor, or the "intelligence information." The result is the waveform shown in Fig. E-3. Note that the amplitude of the carrier is modulated in a symmetrical fashion—i.e., both the positive and negative "envelopes" of the carrier are

165

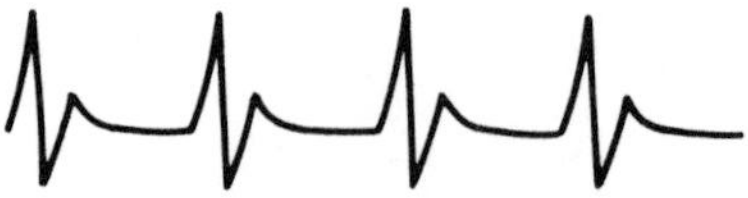

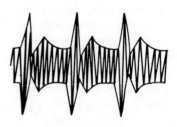

Fig. E-1   Typical heartbeat waveform.

replicas of the impressed waveform. This system is called an amplitude-modulated or AM telemetry system. At the receiver the carrier is picked up by a receiving antenna, amplified, demodulated, and usually presented at an oscilloscope, where a replica of the impressed waveform can be observed.

A system that has gained more popularity recently is frequency-modulated or FM telemetry. A block diagram of a typical FM telemetry system is shown in Fig. E-5.

The unmodulated carrier waveform for an FM telemetry system is identical to that shown in Fig. E-2. The modulated FM waveform, unlike its AM counterpart, does not show any change in carrier amplitude; it does, however, show a change in frequency in accordance with the amplitude of the impressed intelligence, as shown in Fig. E-6.

Referring again to the block diagram of Fig. E-5, it will be seen that the sensor and amplifier portion of the system are those already discussed in the AM system; the amplified signal is fed to a voltage-controlled oscillator (VCO), which generates a frequency-modulated carrier and feeds it to a transmitting antenna. The carrier is received at the receiving antenna, amplified by a radio-frequency amplifier, and fed via a limiter eliminating any incidental amplitude variations to a discriminator, which converts the frequency variations of the FM carrier into the original intelligence signal; that signal is then fed to an oscilloscope for further observation or interpretation and/or recorded on a chart recorder.

Wearers of cardiac telemetry transmitters are usually patients who have just gotten up from the sick bed and are permitted to walk in the hospital

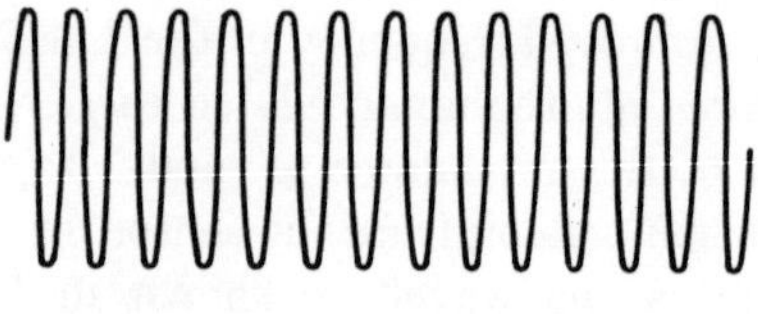

Fig. E-2   Unmodulated carrier.   **Fig. E-3**   Modulated carrier.

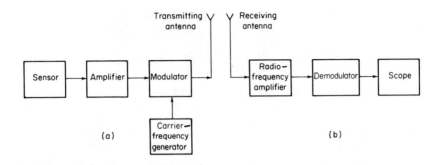

Fig. E-4 Block diagram of typical AM EKG telemetry system. (a) Transmitter. (b) Receiver.

for further observation. It is not unusual for such a patient to develop another heart attack, perhaps due to the strain of walking, or from some other cause; in such an eventuality, prompt action is indicated, often requiring that the patient be quickly defibrillated. There may not even be enough time to remove the cardiac telemetry transmitter attached to the patient, or the nurses and other attendants may simply forget to remove the transmitter prior to such defibrillation attempts. For this reason most modern cardiac telemetry transmitters are built to withstand the voltages produced by defibrillators without any damage to the transmitter itself.

Optical isolation systems employ amplitude modulation; electrodes attached to the patient pick up the patient's heartbeat, the heartbeat is amplified in an amplifier and made to amplitude-modulate a light. The resulting amplitude-modulated light beam impinges on a light-sensitive diode, converting the amplitude-modulated light signal to an equivalent electrical signal, which is further amplified and then displayed on a scope or recorder. The fastest rate at which an optical system, or for that matter any other system, such as an amplifier, can follow abrupt changes of an input signal is called the slew rate. In the case of a step input, i.e. an input which changes its value from a zero or low level to a high level, or from a high level to a zero or low level, the time required to move from 10% to 90% of the final level is called the system's rise and fall time respectively.

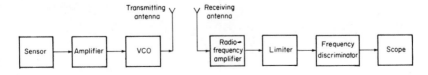

Fig. E-5 Block diagram of typical FM EKG telemetry system.

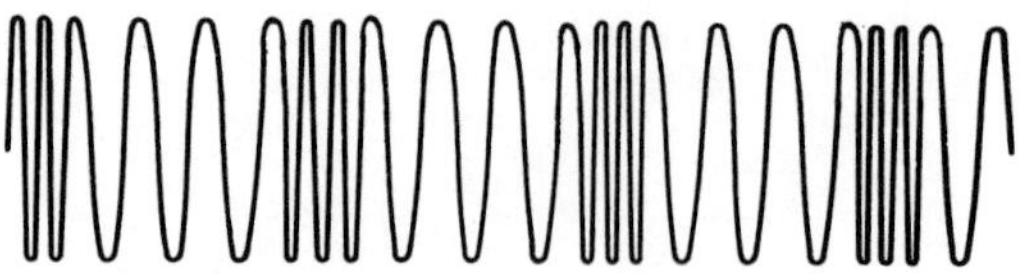

Fig. E-6   Modulated FM carrier.

Modern light modulators and detectors have, as a rule, very short rise and fall times, so that their ability to faithfully follow the EKG waveform does not, generally, present a problem. An optical isolation system has the advantage of isolating a patient from the hospital electrical system while observing or recording instruments permit observation of his EKG waveform.

Cardiac telemetry, however, is almost invariably an FM system; a radio wave, when propagating, is subject to uncontrolled amplitude fluctuations, since it may encounter various obstacles in its path from the transmitter to the receiver. Although such fluctuations, which are usually slow compared to the intelligence signal, can be largely removed by a feature called automatic gain control (AGC) employed in the receiver, it is usually preferable to employ FM for short distances. The limiter incorporated in the FM receiver removes any incidental amplitude modulation of the signal, unless the amplitude of the received carrier falls below the threshold of the limiter. Since the intelligence of an FM signal lies in its frequency variation, amplitude fluctuations due to ordinary propagation conditions will not influence the demodulation process or the shape of the demodulated signal.

Appendix F

EXAMPLE OF ESPA WIRING TO
NFPA STANDARDS

The layout of an ESPA includes a patient reference grounding bus to which all other grounds are connected. Within the patient surroundings, wiring may be fixed to metallic equipment, may be wired as part of the electrical power system, or may be connected by means of patch cords. Each equipment will be grounded according to one of these three techniques, but each method may be used many times in a given installation. The arrangement is shown in Fig. F-1, wherein each method is shown only once for simplicity. In Fig. F-1a, the NFPA requirements are noted on each path. These are the allowable limits listed in Table 4-3. Point A represents the patient reference grounding bus, the central point for all grounding for a given patient. Another patient may share this bus, or he may be tied to another patient reference grounding bus. No patient, however, will be connected to more than one patient reference grounding bus. The power receptacles surrounding the patient location (B) are connected to the bus, permitting electrical instruments to be well-grounded by way of the U-ground connection in the receptacles. Portable devices not requiring electric power may be connected to the bus by use of a patch cable (C), or fixed points such as the bed may be connected by a solid connection (D). The bus itself is connected to the room reference grounding bus (E) by a single wire, which becomes the link to grounds outside of the locale and to structure ground.

In Fig. F-1b, the allowable limits for wire length and size are translated into resistance values. No allowance is made for contact resistance, which is assumed to consist of penetrating contacts, except for the patch cord, which includes an allowance of 0.005 ohm for each plug/jack connection.

One of the critical NFPA requirements states that no ground shall have more than 0.05-ohm resistance from the room reference grounding bus. This means that an acceptable installation must meet the 0.05-ohm limits

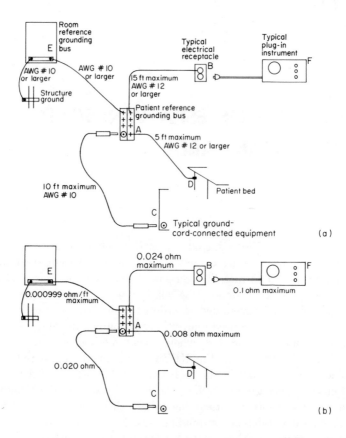

Fig. F-1 (a) Wire length and size limitations in ESPA. (b) Nominal resistance between controlled points *A, B, C, D* in patient area and point *E* outside patient area.

from E to A, B, C, and D, respectively. Two methods are available for controlling this quantity. One consists of controlling the wire-run length from E to A. To hold the total resistance to below 0.05 ohm requires that the length of EA not exceed 26 ft, if AWG # 10 wire is used. For a 26-ft length, the resistance EA is (from Table 4-1) 26 × 0.000999 = 0.026 ohm, and that, added to the resistance of AB just reaches the limit of 0.05 ohms.

When this approach proves inadequate because a longer wire run is needed from E to A, the wire size is enlarged. For example, using AWG #6 wire from E to A permits that length to be increased to 66 ft. The wire resistance of AWG #6 is 0.000395 ohm/ft from Table 4-1, which at 66 ft yields 66 × 0.000395 = 0.026 ohm. It is also possible to gain some advantage by using a larger wire size for run AB, but the improvement thus obtainable is limited because the patch cords quickly become the limiting resistance values for the installation. Patch cords are standardized to AWG #10, and improvements in resistance value can be achieved only by shortening them to less than 10 ft. A length of 6 ft is about as short as is usable in practice, and such a cord has a resistance of 0.012 ohm. Adding the contact resistance of 2 × 0.005 ohm yields a total patch-cord value of 0.017 ohm. Under this condition, the wire lead EA may be made long enough to reach 0.033 ohm, but some allowance should be made for imperfect connections. This limits the length of EA to a value below that computed solely on the basis of wire resistance (typically by 5–20 ft).

It is worthwhile to examine how the installation is protected when a fault occurs. This is shown in Fig. F-2. An instrument plugged into a wall

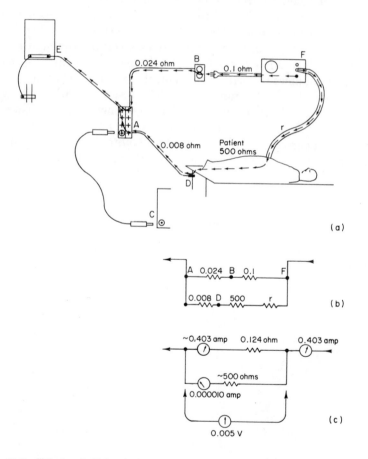

Fig. F-2 Effects of 40.3-mA fault current. (a) Dual path taken by current. (b) Branch through patient has much larger resistance, thus diverting most of the current around patient. (c) Actual current in each branch and voltage on patient.

socket is assumed to develop a fault condition by which some of the power-line current flows into the ground connection at the instrument. As seen in Fig. F-2a, the fault current returns to the power source by two paths, one of which leads through the patient. Each path has a different resistance value, measured from the fault point F to A. The path via the installation ground has a very small resistance value, not exceeding $0.1 + 0.024$ ohm, while the body path has at least the body resistance of, perhaps, 500 ohms. The two paths are shown, in terms of resistances, in Fig. F-2b. The value of r is not known and controlled, but since the conductor is metallic, the resistance is not likely to be significantly large as compared to the body resistance of the patient.

The actual leakage current is, of course, not known in advance. According to NFPA, the objectives of the installation are to keep voltage drops within grounds to less than 0.005 V. The leakage current required to reach this limit is shown in Fig. F-2c. When 0.403 amp emanates from the instrument, the voltage AF reaches 0.005 V. Of the 0.403 amp, only a small fraction, 10 μA, flows through the patient, the remaining current bypassing him by way of the installation ground. The 10-μA current in the patient is presently deemed safe for humans. That a voltage drop no greater than 0.005 V occurs should be verified for all ground points in the patient environment, but from Fig. F-2a it should be quite apparent that no fault voltage larger than that on AF appears on other ground points.

Appendix G

CURRENT LIMITERS

The principles underlying two types of current limiters, the resistance–diode type and the field-effect-diode type, have been presented in Chapter 5. This appendix provides additional circuit details.

Resistance–Diode Limiters

The basic circuit for a grounded-patient-lead current limiter providing protection from both directions was given earlier, in Fig. 5-3b. This circuit is again shown in Fig. G-1a, where the components, currents, and voltages have been identified. When an internal fault voltage occurs in an instrument, this voltage appears across terminals 1–1' or 2–2' of the current limiter. The resulting current flow causes diodes CR_1 and CR_2 to conduct. When the fault is of sufficient magnitude, the diodes reach their maximum voltage, the forward drop of 0.7 V (for silicon). The following treatment assumes that such full conduction is taking place.

The same illustration may be used to gain an understanding of balanced circuits such as those in Fig. 5-3c. One may do this by computing the performance for the ungrounded circuit and then dividing the values obtained for R_1 and R_2 by 2. Within unbalanced circuits, two resistors are then used, having values $R_1/2$ and $R_2/2$, respectively, at the input and output sides.

With diodes CR_1 and CR_2 conducting, the maximum voltage to which a patient will be exposed cannot exceed 0.7 V. By using two reverse-connected diodes, this protection is extended to include faults with negative and positive current components. Additional current limiting by proper selection of R_1 is required to ensure that the patient current can never

173

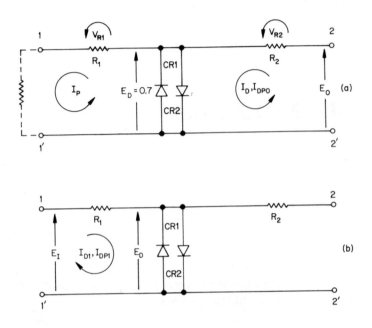

Fig. G-1 Fault currents in resistance–diode current limiter. (a) Fault at 2–2′. (b) Fault at 1–1′.

exceed some predetermined level. For the examples given here, the limit has been selected to be 10 μA.

When a large overvoltage is applied either at input 1–1′ or output 2–2′, the current through diodes CR_1 and CR_2 may well exceed their maximum allowable limits. Since burnout and subsequent loss of protection could result, resistances R_1 and R_2 must be selected properly to avoid this condition. Thus, at least one of these resistances, that on the patient side, serves two functions. One is to protect the patient by limiting the maximum possible current to within safe, predetermined limits; the other is to protect the diodes against burnout (while the patient is not connected). The resistances must also meet two other requirements. Their power ratings must not be exceeded for any of the likely faults anticipated, and their voltage ratings must be adequate for the largest fault voltages that might appear across them.

Consider first a fault originating at terminal 2–2′ while the patient is connected to terminal 1–1′. Assuming that the fault is large enough to cause full diode conduction, voltage E_D becomes 0.7 V and the voltage on the patient side of the diodes can never exceed that value. The actual current through the patient is I_p, controlled by the choice of R_1.

It is also possible to have a fault develop at terminals 1–1′, in which case the roles of R_1 and R_2 become interchanged. R_1 must then be capable of withstanding the fault voltage, while R_2 limits the current out of terminal 2–2′. When this terminal pair is connected to a patient, the same considerations previously discussed for R_1 apply, but to R_2. When the output is an instrument, the value of R_2 is selected to prevent malfunctions. It is not uncommon to require the current limiter to meet both conditions of operation simultaneously, in which event the values of R_1 and R_2 are selected to withstand the more severe conditions.

Table G-1 shows a typical design sequence giving protection against two severe fault types—application of 115-V ac power, and a defibrillation pulse. These two types were chosen as being representative of the most severe conditions likely to be met within the hospital environment. This table shows the design formulas and computations and assumes that a

Table G-1
Sample Computation for Resistance–Diode Current Limiter

1. Find R_2 for 115 V on 2–2′
$$R_2 \approx \frac{E_0}{I_D} = \frac{115}{0.0222} = 5180 \text{ ohms}$$

2. Power dissipated in R_2
$$P_{R2} \approx I_D{}^2 R_2 = (0.0222)^2(5180) = 2.56 \text{ W}$$

3. Find R_1 for 10-μA patient protection
$$R_1 \approx \frac{E_D}{I_p} = \frac{0.7}{10 \times 10^{-6}} = 70,000 \text{ ohms}$$

4. Power dissipated in R_1
$$P_{R1} \approx I_p{}^2 R_1 = (10 \times 10^{-6})^2(70,000) = 7 \times 10^{-6} \text{ W}$$

5. Power dissipated in R_1 for 115 V on 1–1′
$$P_{R1} \approx \frac{E_1{}^2}{R_1} = \frac{(115)^2}{70,000} = 1.89 \text{ W}$$

6. Peak diode current with 800-V pulse 10 msec every 3 sec at 2–2′
$$I_{DPO} \approx \frac{E_0}{R_2} = \frac{800}{5180} = 0.1545 \text{ amp}$$

7. Power dissipated in R_2
$$P_{R2} \approx \frac{(E_0)^2 d}{R_2} = \frac{(800)^2(0.010/3)}{5180} = 0.411 \text{ W}$$

8. Same pulse to 1–1′
$$I_{DPI} \approx \frac{E_1}{R_1} = \frac{800}{70,000} = 0.01144 \text{ amp}$$

9. Power dissipated in R_1
$$P_{R1} \approx \frac{(E_1{}^2)d}{R_1} = \frac{(800)^2(0.010/3)}{70,000} = 0.0305 \text{ amp}$$

specific set of diodes was chosen in advance, having the following characteristics:

maximum continuous current: 20 mA

short-term peak current: 200 mA

These values are representative of commercially available devices. When ac appears due to a fault, only one-half cycle conducts through each diode; the current rating is therefore modified slightly so that an ac current of 22.2 mA becomes equivalent to a continuous dc current of 20 mA.

The results of the table may be summarized as follows: Component R_1 has its ohmic value determined in step 3, its power rating in step 5, and its voltage rating in step 8. Component R_2 has both its ohmic and power ratings determined in step 2 and its voltage rating in step 6. Note that each component undergoes different stresses for each assumed condition. Thus, the selection of such components must be based upon the most severe stress computed.

Resistances R_1 and R_2 tend to have an adverse effect upon the signal levels normally transmitted, especially when the usable signals are naturally small, as with EKG signals. For a 1-mV rms EKG signal, the total resistance of 75,180 ohms reduces the signal current to 13.3 nanoamperes. It is difficult to amplify such a small signal current without adding considerable noise; although more EKG current would be available if R_1 were reduced, this cannot be safely accomplished when using a resistance–diode configuration only. Field-effect diodes, however, make this possible.

Field-Effect-Diode Limiters

The basic circuit for the grounded-patient-lead field-effect-diode current limiter is shown in Fig. 5-4b. This circuit is again given in Fig. G-2, where the components have been identified and the currents and voltages are labeled. Either field-effect diodes or transistors may be used for F_1 and F_2. When a transistor is used, two of the terminals—the source* and the gate—are tied together. The device then acts just like a diode and will be treated as such. Commercially available field-effect diodes seldom have a sufficiently small maximum-current rating to afford adequate patient protection. Adequately rated field-effect transistors, on the other hand, are readily available.

---

* Source, gate and drain are the terminal designations of field-effect transistors, just as emitter, base, and collector are on junction transistors.

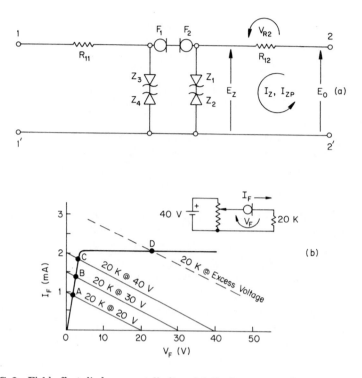

Fig. G-2 Field-effect-diode current limiter. (a) Fault currents. (b) Typical device characteristic.

Placed in series with the signal line, the field-effect diode behaves as shown in Fig. G-2b. As the voltage is increased, the operating point (the point representing the existing voltage and current) follows along a path traversing A, B, and C. With a severe overvoltage, the device operates above the knee of the curve, as at D, where current is essentially constant. In terms of the device resistance, the region below the knee of the curve represents a small resistance level, perhaps 1000 ohms, and it is in this region that normal signal conduction takes place. Above the knee, the dynamic resistance is much higher, often reaching values above 1,000,000 ohms. This characteristic makes the field-effect-diode circuit superior to the resistance–diode type.

The circuits used with field-effect diodes differ from the earlier resistance–diode circuits in two ways: the original resistor R_1 has been replaced by two back-to-back field-effect diodes, and the parallel diodes have been replaced by two back-to-back zener diodes. A zener diode has characteristics similar to those shown in Fig. 5-2, but is operated in a different manner by applying the voltage in reverse to that conventionally applied to diodes. Thus, in the figure, operation is in the lower left region where the voltage is essentially constant regardless of current. The use of zener diodes permits much larger signals to be handled through the current limiter than was heretofore possible with conventional diodes. Zener diodes are readily available in the 2–10-V range, permitting the device to be used in many BMI applications.

In this circuit, the zener diodes act as protective devices for the field-effect diodes by preventing a voltage buildup to values large enough to exceed the field-effect-diode voltage ratings. The zener diodes, in turn, are protected from the application of excessive power by resistances R_{11} and R_{12}.

Table G-2 shows a typical design sequence giving protection against the same faults previously applied to the resistance–diode circuit. It is assumed that the field-effect diodes are initially chosen with a constant-current rating satisfying the maximum safe patient-current requirements and that their resistances are 1000 ohms. The zener diodes are assumed to be the 5-V types, having a maximum continuous current rating of 40 mA and a short-term peak current rating of 800 mA.

The results may be summarized as follows. Both R_{11} and R_{12} are chosen on the same basis, and their values and ratings will be the same. The ohmic values are obtained in step 1, the power ratings in step 2, and the voltage ratings in step 3.

Table G-2
Sample Computation for Field-Effect-Diode Current Limiter

1. Find R_{12} for 115 V on 2–2′

$$R_{12} \approx \frac{E_0 - E_z}{I_z} = \frac{115 - 5}{40 \times 10^{-3}} = 2740 \text{ ohms}$$

2. Power dissipated in R_{12}

$$P_{R12} \approx \frac{(E_0 - E_z)^2}{R_{12}} = \frac{(115 - 5)^2}{2740} = 4.4 \text{ W}$$

3. Peak zener current with 800-V pulse 10 msec every 3 sec at 2–2′

$$I_{zp} \approx \frac{E_0 - E_z}{R_{12}} = \frac{800 - 5}{2740} = 0.29 \text{ amp}$$

4. Power dissipated in R_{12}

$$P_{R12} \approx \frac{(E_0 - E_z)^2 d}{R_{12}} = \frac{(800 - 5)^2(0.010/3)}{2740} = 0.769 \text{ W}$$

5. Values for R_{11}

Same as for R_{12}

The total circuit resistance presented to a transmitted signal is now 6480 ohms and, for an EKG signal of 1 mV rms, the current flow is 154 nA. This current level is much more compatible with the input needs of EKG instruments than the earlier 13.3 nAm and ensures a more stable, more reliable, and less noisy data transfer. It may be noted that patient safety was not sacrificed to improved performance, the only cost penalty being a few more electronic components.

Appendix H

VOLTAGE–SENSING GROUND MONITORS

The purposes and basic operating principles of several ground monitors were presented in the main text. One of these, the voltage-sensing type, is widely used. This appendix provides the following additional information concerning these devices.

1. It defines the criteria for an ideal ground monitor to which practical devices may be compared.
2. It shows the limitations inherent in practical devices.
3. It gives performance measures for practical devices.
4. It shows how performance may be optimized.

The Ideal Ground Monitor

It is desirable to establish at the start a set of ideal relationships that one would wish to obtain in a particular device. These ideals will then form a basis for comparison with actual devices, will show how closely the ideal is approached and what are the shortcomings of practical devices. The nature of the hazard for which protection is required must necessarily determine what the ideal ground monitor should be like. For example, in an environment of flammable anesthetics, any occurrence of a spark could be disastrous. Thus, for this application, the ideal ground monitor will detect every potential condition that might result in sparking, including all faults from power lines to ground. The detector that will sound the alarm, however, does not monitor the power-line currents but measures instead a current flow through the detector into ground. The two currents—the fault current and the detector current—are not the same. Ideally, they

180

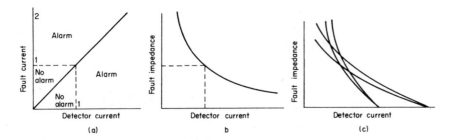

Fig. H-1 Detector characteristics. (a) and (b) Ideal. (c) Representative of the different curves applying to varying fault types.

should relate so that an increase in fault current causes a proportional increase in detector current. Or alternatively, the detector current should decrease with fault impedance. These two ideal relationships are shown in Fig. H-1. We are specifically interested in one point along the curves, that value of fault impedance or fault current at which the alarm should be activated.

In practice, it is impossible to attain the proportional relationships shown. Instead, various faults may result in different curves, typically as shown in Fig. H-1c. Unless all the curves can be made to intersect at just one point, the alarm will not be activated each time at the same fault current and impedance. Practical systems fall short of these requirements. Instead of activating the alarm at a predetermined value of fault current and impedance, they activate it at a specific value of detector current. Then, depending upon the nature of the fault—resistive or capacitive— this alarm point may correspond to different amounts of fault current and impedance.

Hazard Indexes

One quantitative measure of the protection afforded by a ground monitor is given by the hazard indexes. The *total hazard index* has two components. One is the *fault hazard index*, which is the upper limit of fault current permitted by the device. This limit may alternatively be stated as a fault impedance (line voltage divided by maximum fault current). Generally, when the limit has been reached, an alarm is activated and some method for disconnecting power may be initiated. The second component is the *detector hazard index*, representing the maximum possible current flow through the detector to ground. This worst condition will occur when one of the power lines is grounded. Taken separately, each of the two components is independent of the nature of the fault which might accidentally occur— i.e., whether the fault impedance is resistive or capacitive.* Although unlikely, these two current components could be simultaneously present in the ground, as shown in Fig. H-2; this combination constitutes the worst-case hazard.

Added together, the two indexes constitute the total hazard index. Although proper addition of currents is performed vectorially (see Chapter 2), the largest and therefore most conservative value of total hazard index is obtained by just adding the two indexes arithmetically. When computed vectorially, the total hazard index varies according to whether the fault is resistive, capacitive, or some combination of resistive and capacitive impedances.

When the detector is used to activate an alarm, it is desirable to know what protection level is actually being afforded before the alarm activates. The indexes mentioned so far do not provide this information. Another measure, the *undetected total hazard index*, does. It also has two components, one of which is the previously described detector hazard index. The second component is the fault current required to just activate the alarm. Both components are added vectorially; their sum will be different for various fault conditions. This variation of fault current is not desirable and constitutes a major shortcoming of the voltage-sensing ground monitor.

Suppose in a given ground monitor, the alarm is set to be activated at a detector current corresponding to a fault current exactly equal to the fault hazard index of the system when the fault is a single pure resistance. Both

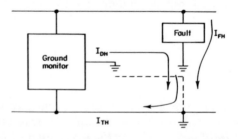

Fig. H-2   Worst-case hazard. One power line accidentally grounded and a fault from the other. I_{DH} is the detector hazard index, I_{FH} the fault hazard index, and I_{TH} the total hazard index.

* Inductive faults are seldom present in practice and are therefore omitted from further discussion.

the total and the undetected total hazard index are then identical. Suppose further that a capacitive rather than resistive fault of the same magnitude occurred. The detector current would then be larger than before, as will be shown in a later example, and the alarm would trip. However, the alarm actually goes off before the fault current has reached the expected magnitude because the detector current rises to the alarm level at a smaller quantity of fault current. Thus, the capacitive fault provides more comprehensive protection than a resistive fault. The undetected total hazard index will then consist of the vectorial sum of the fault current at alarm and the detector hazard index. Alternatively, a fault might occur for which the detector current never reaches the threshold value. The fault then remains undetected, and the undetected total hazard index becomes infinite. Ground monitors operating in a blind spot behave this way.

A numerical example will serve to illustrate hazard indexes. Consider the detector in Fig. H-3a. It consists of three resistances. Assuming that protection is desired against faults under 60,000 ohms, the fault index is determined by the ratio of line voltage to resistance, or $120/60,000 = 2$ mA. In order to make the computation easier, the circuit in Fig. H-3a is first converted into its equivalent circuit in Fig. H-3b using Thévenin's theorem. As far as any load is concerned at a–a', the currents in and out of a–a' are identical among the circuits in Figs. H-3a and H-3b, and so are the voltages across a–a' (see Chapter 2). The detector has a hazard current of its own, corresponding to the detector current when one power line is grounded. This condition is obtained by connecting a to a'. The detector hazard index is 1 mA and the total hazard index is 3 mA. So far, the detector current at which the alarm is to be activated, has not been chosen. Later, it will be shown that the choice is not completely arbitrary. For now, let us assume that the alarm is activated at a fault current of 2 mA for a single resistive fault. Figure H-3c shows that the alarm current is 0.5 mA. (The alarm system is presumed to be included in the 30-K resistance shown in Fig. H-3a). Once the alarm level is set, regardless of fault type, whenever the detector current reaches 0.5 mA, the alarm will activate. Because of our choice, both undetected total and total hazard index are the same.

When the same 60-K fault impedance, this time capacitive, is introduced, as in Fig. H-3d, the fault current is again 2 mA. The detector current, however, is now 0.707mA, which is above the threshold for alarm set at 0.5 mA. It actually activates the alarm long before the detector current reaches 0.707 mA. The corresponding fault impedance at alarm is no longer 60 K but a much larger impedance, 104 K, shown in Fig. H-3e. But when the fault impedance is 104 K, the fault current is only 1.155 mA which, combined vectorially with the detector hazard index of 1 mA,

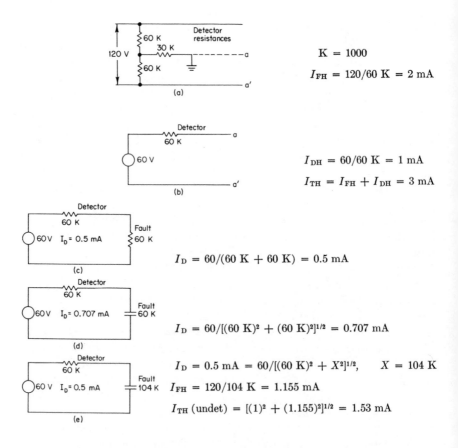

$K = 1000$

$I_{FH} = 120/60\ K = 2$ mA

$I_{DH} = 60/60\ K = 1$ mA

$I_{TH} = I_{FH} + I_{DH} = 3$ mA

$I_D = 60/(60\ K + 60\ K) = 0.5$ mA

$I_D = 60/[(60\ K)^2 + (60\ K)^2]^{1/2} = 0.707$ mA

$I_D = 0.5$ mA $= 60/[(60\ K)^2 + X^2]^{1/2}$, $\qquad X = 104\ K$

$I_{FH} = 120/104\ K = 1.155$ mA

I_{TH} (undet) $= [(1)^2 + (1.155)^2]^{1/2} = 1.53$ mA

Fig. H-3   Hazard indexes. Computational example.

yields an undetected total hazard index of 1.53mA. Thus, the capacitive fault gives a different value for undetected total hazard index from that for the resistive fault, and for the capacitive fault 1.53 mA represents the maximum hazard present prior to alarm. These differences indicate the variations of protection to be expected from voltage-sensing ground monitors. The specific faults illustrated here are representative of a multitude of other fault types, which must all be taken into account if the ground monitor is to be properly assessed. For this reason, the behavior of ground monitors under a variety of fault types will be further discussed in this appendix beginning on p. 189.

Before proceeding, however, it is worthwhile to examine some of the internal characteristics of voltage-sensing ground monitors necessary for proper performance. This examination will show that it will be necessary to impose some restrictions on the values and types of internal components of the monitor.

Internal Characteristics of Ground Monitors

The detector circuit of Fig. H-4 is commonly used for ground monitors. The specific performance attainable from the detector will depend upon the choice of component values within the detector. It is reasonable to expect that the detector current ought to be the same whether a fault occurs from one power line or the other, and this consideration determines the relationship between Z_1 and Z_2 as follows.

1. The detector impedance shall be the same from one power line as from the other, to ensure equal detection sensitivity to the same fault from either line.

Impedances Z_1 and Z_2 may be resistive, capacitive, or in combination, but in order to ensure that the detector is equally sensitive to resistive and capacitive faults, the detection circuit must be so arranged that the current flow in either case is the same. This can be ensured by making the resistive component of total detection impedance equal to its capacitive reactance; any circuit meeting this condition has an impedance phase angle of $-45°$. It follows that:

2. The overall detector impedance shall have a phase angle of $-45°$, to ensure equal sensitivity to purely resistive and purely capacitive faults.

In this connection, total impedance consists of Z_1 and Z_2, considered to be connected in parallel, and added to Z_5, as may be seen from the equivalent circuit in Fig. H-4b. How equal sensitivity is achieved by these rules is shown in Fig. H-5, where the total detector impedance has been replaced by a resistance R_D and a capacitive reactance X_D.

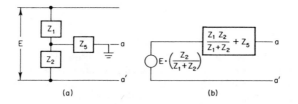

Fig. H-4 Ground monitor. (a) and (b) Equivalent circuits so far as output a–a′ is concerned.

It was noted earlier that the bridge circuit has a blind spot for which no current flows in the central leg. It was also noted that the blind spot occurs when the voltages developed across the lower impedances of the bridge just balance (voltages ac as compared to bc in Fig. 5-8a). When used as a ground monitor, the center leg of the bridge appears in effect from the mid-point of the detector to the ground point of the fault. But the midpoint assumes exactly the value of voltage and phase of the Thévenin equivalent-circuit voltage source in Fig. H-4, and therefore the bridge will balance when the ground point of the fault assumes exactly that voltage and phase. It follows that:

3.   All *static* detectors have blind spots, consisting of some combination of fault impedances, connected from each power line to ground, that will cause the detector current to drop to zero, even though a line fault is actually present.

Since the blind spot for any given bridge circuit occurs at just one particular point, namely the point at which the fault voltage equals the equivalent-circuit source voltage of the detector both in magnitude and phase, there can be just one fault combination at which the blind spot occurs (and, of course, circuits that are electrically equivalent). It is possible, therefore, to arrange the circuit in such a manner that two voltage sources are present, with different equivalent values. The dynamic detector accomplishes this goal by switching, alternately, from one voltage source to another. It is true that each sample, taken individually, can experience

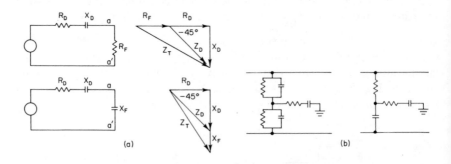

(a)   (b)

Fig. H-5   45° Detector impedance. (a) Total impedance Z_T has same absolute value for resistive or capacitive fault. (b) Two circuits capable of providing 45° detector impedance. When equivalent detector impedance has equally resistive and reactive components R_D and X_D, the total impedance Z_D is at $-45°$. The faults add to the vectors in line with either R_D or X_D. In either case, as long as Z_D is at $-45°$, equal faults R_F or X_F result in a vector of the same total length Z_T. Hence, detector current is the same for either fault.

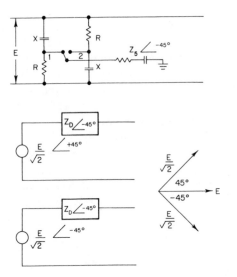

Fig. H-6 Dynamic detector, equally sensitive to resistance and capacitance, having no blind spot. By setting $X = R$, the detector impedance is at $-45°$. The equivalent voltage source is $E/\sqrt{2}$ in both switch positions 1 and 2, but the phase angle switches from $+45°$ to $-45°$. This is shown in the phasor diagram.

a blind spot, but the blind spots of the two samples cannot coincide as long as the two voltage sources differ in value. Therefore:

4. A *dynamic* detector cannot have a blind spot, as long as the two voltage sources differ in magnitude, phase, or both.

A suitable dynamic detector circuit is shown in Fig. H-6. This circuit has an equivalent impedance of $-45°$ and its voltage source alternates between $+45°$ and $-45°$ with respect to line voltage. As a result, although both voltage sources are numerically identical, their phase angles are different, one being $+45°$ and the other $-45°$. Hence, the blind spot for one circuit cannot be simultaneously present for the other, so that some detector current will flow for all fault conditions.

Detector Amplitude Characteristics

In a dynamic detector, two voltages, sampled independently, need to be combined, and there are various ways of doing this. The method chosen may even provide an opportunity to improve detector performance.

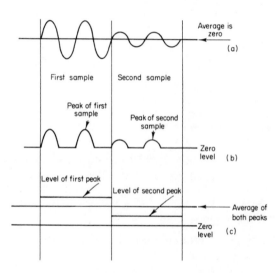

The detection process takes place as shown in Fig. H-7. Since the average value of an ac waveform is zero, the two signals are first rectified by removing the negative portion of each signal. The detector then notes the maximum signal in each of the two sampling intervals. At this point, a choice is made as to how to combine the signals from each sampling interval. Figure H-7d shows the rules applying to three types of detectors— peak, average, and quasi-peak detectors.

Whenever the signals sampled in each interval are of the same magnitude, all the detectors behave alike. Thus, the differences relating to the specific detector chosen arise only when the two samples differ. Thus, the choice of a type of detector bears only on those fault conditions that result in differences between the two samples. With the quasi-peak detector,

Type of detector	Output level
Peak	Highest peak among both samples
Average	Average of both peaks
Quasi-peak	Intermediate between peak and average
	Factor a lies between $a = 1$ for average and $a = 2$ for peak
	Then, detector current is
	$I_{QP} = I_{av} + a\,(I_{pk} - I_{av})$ (d)

Fig. H-7 Detector characteristics. The ac waveform (a) is rectified in (b) and the peak value of each sample is noted (c). Three detectors use this waveform as shown in (d).

the constant a may be selected to improve overall performance, as will be shown later.

5. The constant a of a quasi-peak detector of a dynamic ground monitor is insensitive to all faults that provide equal current samples, and it may be selected to compensate perfectly for some specific fault types for which the detection-current samples differ.

Detector Behavior for Various Fault Types

Faults may consist of resistances or capacitances, singly or in combination, from power line to ground or between power lines. Faults between power lines are not detected by the ground monitor. Leakage currents from equipments to ground are not true faults, but the ground monitor sees them exactly as if they were faults. Because they are indistinguishable from true faults, they will be treated as faults.

Faults may be *single*, from one power line to ground, or *multiple*, occurring simultaneously from both power lines. For example, when a leakage path exists from one power line and a true fault develops from the other power line, a multiple fault is considered to be present. In the most general case, the impedances from one power line differ from those from the other. An exception to these *unbalanced faults* occurs when both impedances are alike. This category is termed the *balanced faults*. The necessity to evaluate the different fault types stems from the earlier observations that the ground detector responds differently to various faults.

In the process of analyzing various faults, the objective is to find ways to minimize performance differences so that every time the alarm is activated, essentially the same hazard is present. The analysis proceeds as follows.

For each fault type, the actual circuit is first converted into a Thévenin equivalent circuit. This new circuit will contain one or two voltage sources as well as the impedances representing the detector and the fault. The current flow computed for the equivalent circuit will be the same as the detector current in the original circuit. Since the quantities of voltage and impedance in an ac circuit add vectorially, the necessary vector diagrams will be shown.* There will be two such diagrams, an impedance diagram and a voltage diagram. The impedance diagram shows how the various components of detector and fault impedances are combined to arrive at a

---

* The vector relationships are all time relationships, with angles representing phase differences in the ac waveforms. Time-related vectors are also known as phasors.

total impedance. The detector-current vector is drawn horizontally facing to the right, and all resistance components are also drawn in this direction. Capacitive components are drawn at an angle of 90°, facing down. When all vectors are proportioned to component magnitude, the total impedance is that vector which completes the triangle. The impedance diagram then yields both the magnitude of the total impedance and its angular relationship (in time) to the detector current. This entire diagram is superimposed upon the voltage diagram so that the total impedance coincides with the equivalent net voltage source vector.

In the voltage diagram, the impedance vectors assume the meaning of voltage drops, each being equal to the product of the detector current and the impedance component shown. Superimposing the total mpedance upon the net voltage source is equivalent to stating that the voltage applied to a series circuit equals the sum of the voltage drops across all the circuit components. For convenience, the power-line voltage E is drawn horizontally facing right. The equivalent voltage sources may differ from E both as to magnitude and phase angle, and these vectors are placed on the diagram accordingly. Such a voltage diagram will show, for each fault type, the magnitude and phase angle of the detector-current vector. However, the detector alarm circuit reacts only to current magnitude. When a dynamic detector is used, each of the two samples yields a different diagram. The procedure is illustrated in Fig. H-8. In a subsequent presentation of the various fault types, the two voltage diagrams in Figs. H-8c and H-8d will, however, be combined into a single diagram.

A. *Single Faults*

The three types of single faults to be presented are the single resistance, the single capacitance, and the combination of one resistance and one capacitance from the same power line to ground when resistance equals capacitive reactance. These three types are shown in Fig. H-9. The dynamic detector used to detect these faults will be that given in Fig. H-6.

B. *Balanced Faults*

The same types of faults are shown again in Fig. H-10, except that each fault is assumed to occur twice simultaneously, once from each power line to ground. The equivalent circuit for balanced faults differs from the earlier circuits by having one additional voltage source present.

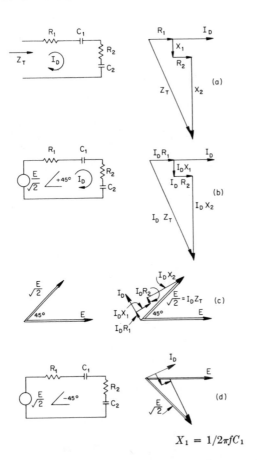

$$X_1 = 1/2\pi f C_1 \qquad X_2 = 1/2\pi f C_2$$

Fig. H-8 Illustration of vector diagrams for fault analysis. (a) Right: Impedance diagram for circuit at left. R_1 and C_1 may represent the detector, R_2 and C_2 the fault. Magnitudes are represented as vector lengths. (b) When a voltage source is connected to the circuit, the resultant voltage drops may be represented by same vector diagram, but relabeled as voltages. (c) Voltage source $(E/\sqrt{2}) \angle 45°$ is first drawn (left), then $I_D Z_T$ and entire impedance diagram is superimposed (right). The diagram shows how detector current I_D relates to line voltage E. (d) Left: in a dynamic detector, the second sample may have a voltage source $(E/\sqrt{2}) \angle -45°$. Right: the resultant diagram is shown. I_D assumes, alternately, the values in (c) and (d).

C. *Equalization*

Considering only the six fault types just shown, best performance would be obtained if, for the same fault impedance, the detector currents were all identical in magnitude. Of the six fault types, only four different detector currents are actually obtained. The detector currents in Figs. H-9a and

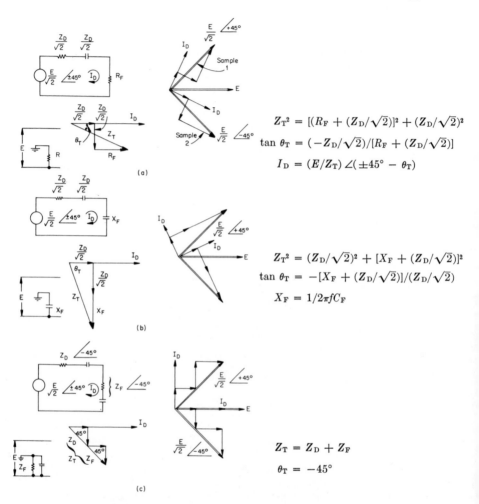

$$Z_T{}^2 = [(R_F + (Z_D/\sqrt{2})]^2 + (Z_D/\sqrt{2})^2$$
$$\tan \theta_T = (-Z_D/\sqrt{2})/[R_F + (Z_D/\sqrt{2})]$$
$$I_D = (E/Z_T) \angle(\pm 45° - \theta_T)$$

(a)

$$Z_T{}^2 = (Z_D/\sqrt{2})^2 + [X_F + (Z_D/\sqrt{2})]^2$$
$$\tan \theta_T = -[X_F + (Z_D/\sqrt{2})]/(Z_D/\sqrt{2})$$
$$X_F = 1/2\pi f C_F$$

(b)

$$Z_T = Z_D + Z_F$$
$$\theta_T = -45°$$

(c)

Fig. H-9 Examples of single faults. (a) Fault is resistance R_F. (b) Fault is capacitive reactance X_F. (c) Fault Z_F is equally resistive and reactive.

H-9b are identical, and so are those in Figs. H-10a and H-10b, as a consequence of following rule 2. Since the detector impedance Z_D enters each expression for the total impedance Z_t, it may be possible to choose Z_D in such a way that two of the four current values can be made to coincide. Variations of the fault impedance at the alarm point can thereby be reduced. Indeed, this equalization is possible. Figure H-11 shows how the fault impedance varies with detector impedance for both single and balanced faults. It is desired to find a point on these curves at which all the

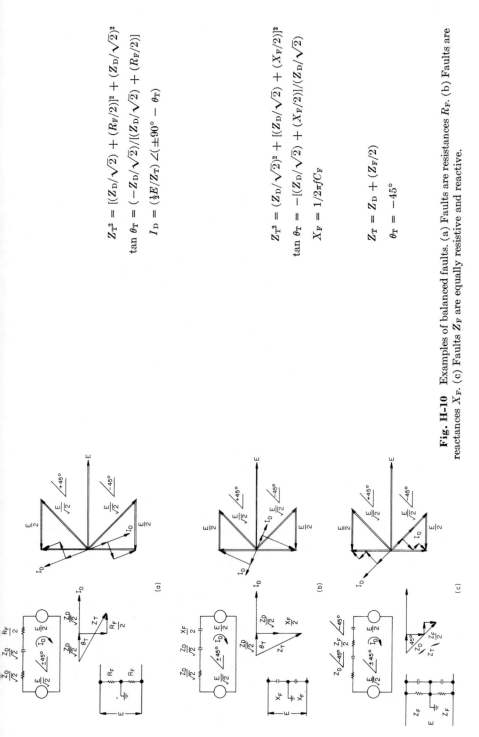

$$Z_T{}^2 = [(Z_D/\sqrt{2}) + (R_F/2)]^2 + (Z_D/\sqrt{2})^2$$

$$\tan \theta_T = (-Z_D/\sqrt{2})/[(Z_D/\sqrt{2}) + (R_F/2)]$$

$$I_D = (\tfrac{1}{2}E/Z_T) \angle (\pm 90° - \theta_T)$$

$$Z_T{}^2 = (Z_D/\sqrt{2})^2 + [(Z_D/\sqrt{2}) + (X_F/2)]^2$$

$$\tan \theta_T = -[(Z_D/\sqrt{2}) + (X_F/2)]/(Z_D/\sqrt{2})$$

$$X_F = 1/2\pi f C_F$$

$$Z_T = Z_D + (Z_F/2)$$

$$\theta_T = -45°$$

Fig. H-10 Examples of balanced faults. (a) Faults are resistances R_F. (b) Faults are reactances X_F. (c) Faults Z_F are equally resistive and reactive.

193

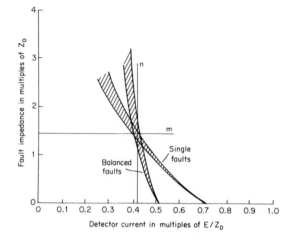

Fig. H-11   Fault-impedance variation with detector impedance.

curves are as close together as possible. This point occurs at the inter-section of lines m and n and corresponds to setting the expressions for the detector current of Figs. H-9c and H-10c equal to each other.

The important conclusion is that equalization among single and balanced faults requires that the detector impedance Z_D be made a fixed percentage of the desired fault impedance at alarm. The required relationship, stated here without proof, is $Z_D = 0.707Z_f$. Once selected, the detector current at alarm is also fully determined to be

$$I_D = 0.414 \ (E/Z_D) = 0.414I_{DH} = 0.586 \ (E/Z_F)$$

The equalization is not perfect because detector current has not been equalized for other than the two fault types described. It may be demon-strated, however, that all fault-impedance variation will remain within 20% among all single and balanced faults.

D.   *Unbalanced Faults*

All faults that are neither single nor balanced are unbalanced faults. This class covers all possible combinations of resistance and capacitance that could occur from both power lines to ground. The equivalent circuit is shown in Fig. H-12. The accompanying vector diagram shows the range of values assumed by the net equivalent voltage source, and these are seen to lie within two circles. The horizontal line through each circle represents all voltage-source vectors for single and balanced faults but also includes some unbalanced faults. All voltage vectors terminating on these lines yield two identical samples from a dynamic detector. Therefore, no fault lying along these lines can be equalized by making use of a specific detector characteristic. Conversely, all faults lying elsewhere within these circles can be so equalized.

To gain a better understanding of the circle diagrams, Fig. H-13 is presented, showing two typical classes of unbalanced faults and their

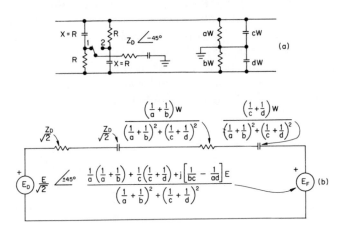

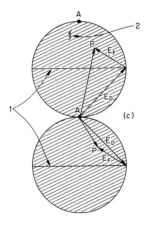

Fig. H-12 General fault formulation. (a) Original circuit. Constants W, a, b, c, d may take on any positive value. (b) Equivalent circuit. (c) Range of phasors. Point 1: The tips P of vectors lie along this line for all faults for which each sample is numerically equal to the other (indifferent to quasi-peak detector constant). Point 2: Shaded regions show where tip P of vector may lie for any fault. Point A shows tip location for which quasi-peak detector constant is often chosen.

equivalent voltage-source locations in the circles. For each type, the equivalent circuit and the voltage vector diagram are shown, with V_c representing the net voltage source. The amount of unbalance varies with a and b, and each individual value of these constants describes a different fault. As a and b vary, so will the voltage source V_c, and a point P shown in the figure moves along a straight line or circular path. A portion of the double circle of Fig. H-12c is also shown. Point P always remains within the double circle. Only one point P can be completely equalized by choosing the constant a of the quasi-peak detector. Most other faults, however, will require a different value of a to be equalized.

The uppermost point in the circle diagram in Fig. H-12c is point A. The fault represented by this point is shown in Fig. H-14. One sample of its dynamic detector operates in the blind spot and thus has no detector current. The other does. The manner in which the two samples are averaged

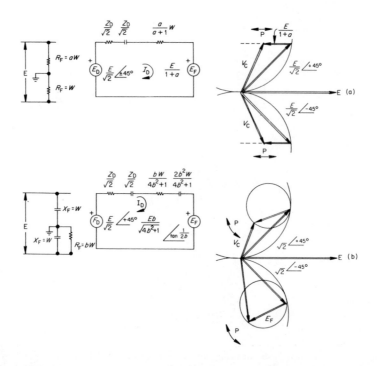

Fig. H-13 Examples of unbalanced faults. (a) Pure resistance faults. As a varies, point P moves along a straight line from the rim through the center of the circle. V_C is voltage across the circuit impedances. (b) Two equal capacitances and a varying resistive fault. As b varies, point P moves along the dashed circle. The two different samples are represented by the two different lengths of V_C.

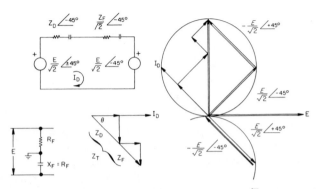

Fig. H-14 Unbalanced fault $R_F = X_F$. $Z_T = Z_D + (Z_F/\sqrt{2})$; $\theta = -45°$. Sample 1, $I_D = (E/Z_T) \angle +135°$. Sample 2, $I_D = 0$.

can be adjusted to make the detector current exactly the same as that obtained for the two faults compensated for earlier, the single and the balanced fault combination of one resistance and one equal capacitive reactance. To do this requires a quasi-peak detector with constant $a = 0.171$.

The fault impedance variation at the alarm point was determined earlier to be no more than 20%, but needs to be modified now to account for unbalanced faults. Additional sources of impedance variation are due to the unbalanced faults lying along the central horizontals within the two circles of Fig. H-12c. The faults include the purely resistive faults of Fig. H-13a and corresponding purely capacitive faults. These can contribute an additional 15% impedance variation at alarm, making the total now 35%.

The fault impedance at alarm can also be expected to vary for all other unbalanced faults. Assuming that these are being equalized at the single point A in Fig. H-12c, no additional impedance variations at alarm will accrue.

Leakage Capacitance and False Alarms

One of the more disturbing problems in connection with ground monitors is the likely occurrence of false alarms—alarm conditions due to ground currents arising, not from faults, but from natural leakage within transformers, cables, and filters. Since they are not indicative of an equipment fault, their occurrence could well be confusing. Activation of the alarm however, means that there exists a significant ground-current flow due to the leakage, and therefore a possible hazard.

The common sources of stray currents are found within the fixed portions of the installation—the isolation transformer, the wiring, the ground monitor—but also in connection with all the equipments plugged into the receptacles. The former can be predetermined for a given installation, or can be measured. Capacitances in this portion usually range from 2000 to 6000 pF, having an impedance at 60-Hz line frequency from 1.33 megohm to 442 kilohms. The larger capacitances are generally associated with the more powerful isolation units. When, in addition, the unpredictable leakage currents of all the plug-in instruments are taken into account, the total impedance due to leakages may well approach the fault-impedance magnitude at which the alarm will normally be activated.

The particular fault type representing the condition of a balanced set of capacitances and an additional possible fault resistance has already been presented in Fig. H-13b. The balanced set of capacitances can represent the leakage currents, and the resistance can simulate the fault. It is of interest to find out how the performance of the ground detector is altered by the presence of the capacitances and, in particular, at what value of fault resistance the alarm will now be activated.

The performance of the dynamic detector discussed previously under these conditions is shown in Fig. H-15. The detector impedance is also assumed to be chosen for best equalization as before. The curve shows the relationship between the amount of leakage present and the value of fault

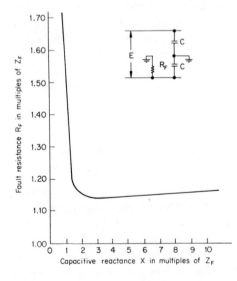

Fig. H-15 Alarm point in the presence of balanced capacitance. Z_F is the design value of fault impedance at alarm, and $X = 1/2\pi f C$.

resistance then required to set off the alarm. All quantities are presented as multiples of the fault impedance for which the ground monitor was designed.

The curve shows that whenever the capacitance is small enough so that its reactance is at least twice the impedance Z_f, the ground detector is substantially unaffected by the presence of the capacitances. In fact, it performs slightly better than if they were absent. With too much capacitance, however, where the capacitive reactance is less than twice the fault impedance, serious false-alarm conditions can exist. For example, when the capacitive reactance just equals the fault impedance, the alarm will activate prematurely for resistive faults. At this point on the curve, $R_F = 1.60 \times Z_F$. A resistive fault, instead of activating the alarm at a fault resistance equal to the fault impedance, actually sets off the alarm at a fault resistance 60% higher.

It may be concluded that careful control over all instruments to be plugged into the installation is necessary to ensure that the total capacitance does not become too large. False-alarm problems can then be avoided.

Appendix I

THREE–RESISTANCE RECEPTACLE TESTING

A brief introductory description of the three-resistance receptacle test technique, wherein a voltmeter gives direct fault indications, is given in the main text. This appendix provides a detailed analysis and shows how the resistances R_1, R_2, and R_3 must be chosen.

The basic circuit and all the equivalent circuits and formulas corresponding to each fault are given in Fig. I-1. Although the circuits are different for various faults, it cannot be assumed that the meter deflections are also different unless the resistance values are chosen with great care. To this end, several observations are significant: three conditions—normal, reversed H–N, and reversed H–G—depend upon all three resistances, while the other two faults—open G and open N—depend only upon two resistances. Furthermore, when we inspect the three former expressions, a

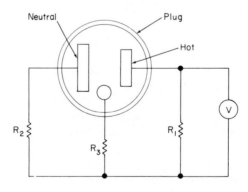

Fig. I-1a

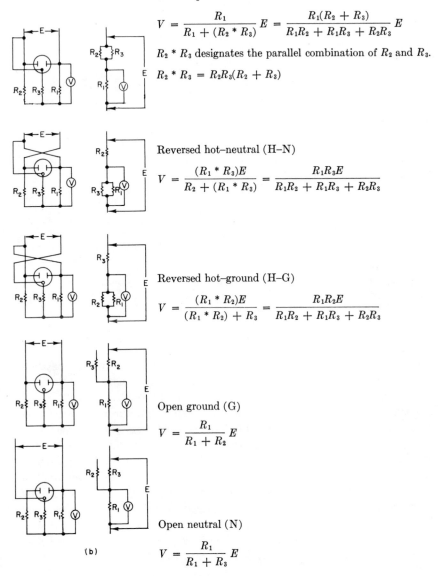

Normal performance

$$V = \frac{R_1}{R_1 + (R_2 * R_3)} E = \frac{R_1(R_2 + R_3)}{R_1 R_2 + R_1 R_3 + R_2 R_3} E$$

$R_2 * R_3$ designates the parallel combination of R_2 and R_3.

$$R_2 * R_3 = R_2 R_3 (R_2 + R_3)$$

Reversed hot–neutral (H–N)

$$V = \frac{(R_1 * R_3)E}{R_2 + (R_1 * R_3)} = \frac{R_1 R_3 E}{R_1 R_2 + R_1 R_3 + R_2 R_3}$$

Reversed hot–ground (H–G)

$$V = \frac{(R_1 * R_2)E}{(R_1 * R_2) + R_3} = \frac{R_1 R_2 E}{R_1 R_2 + R_1 R_3 + R_2 R_3}$$

Open ground (G)

$$V = \frac{R_1}{R_1 + R_2} E$$

Open neutral (N)

$$V = \frac{R_1}{R_1 + R_3} E$$

(b)

Fig. I-1 Diagnostic testing of receptacles by the three-resistance technique. (a) Basic circuit. (b) Equivalent circuits and output for normal performance and for various fault conditions.

$$\frac{\text{Reversed hot–neutral}}{\text{Normal}} = \frac{R_1 R_3}{R_1 R_2 + R_1 R_3} = \frac{1}{1 + (R_2/R_3)}$$

$$\frac{\text{Reversed hot–ground}}{\text{Normal}} = \frac{R_1 R_2}{R_1 R_2 + R_1 R_3} = \frac{1}{1 + (R_3/R_2)} = 1 - \frac{1}{1 + (R_2/R_3)}$$

(a)

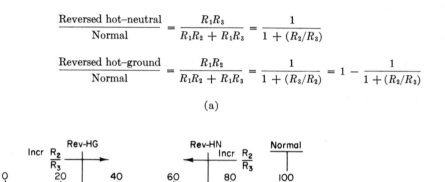

(b)

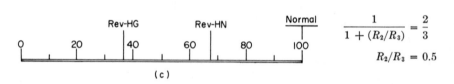

$$\frac{1}{1 + (R_2/R_3)} = \frac{2}{3}$$

$$R_2/R_3 = 0.5$$

(c)

Fig. I-2 Interrelationship of normal, reversed H–N, and reversed H–G measurements. (a) Ratio of indications obtained. (b) Indications as R_2 is varied. (c) Most favorable indications for which $R_2/R_3 = 0.5$.

common denominator is observed, which suggests that if we divide these expressions among themselves, simpler relationships may be obtainable. Indeed this is true, and the relationships are shown in Fig. I-2a. As an illustration of these relationships, let us assume that the meter reads 100 under normal conditions. Both the reversed H–N and the reversed H–G readings will then always be less than 100, but they will always be such that the sum of the reversed H–N and the reversed H–G readings is exactly 100. They could thus be 50/50 or 30/70 or some other combination determined by the ratio R_2/R_3. An instrument reading of 50/50 would not distinguish the two faults, making it necessary to choose R_2/R_3 so that this condition is avoided. It seems most reasonable to divide the scale equally among the faults. This is achieved by making the ratio of reversed H–G to reversed H–N 33.3/66.7, as shown in Fig. 1-2c. For this condition, $R_2/R_3 = 0.5$.

With this ratio chosen, we now embark upon the selection process for R_1 so that the other faults, no G and no N, appear as nonoverlapping meter deflections. We illustrate the problem by the curves in Fig. I-3, where the ratio R_3/R_1 is varied while holding $R_2/R_3 = 0.5$. The scale at the left is the fraction of the line voltage registered by the voltmeter under these conditions. The most evenly spaced conditions are obtained near $R_3/R_1 =$ 2.8. Thus, all the required conditions for separating faults by unique meter deflections can be met, even though the resistance R_1 has not been specifically selected. For any R_1, however, both R_2 and R_3 are predetermined by the ratios $R_2/R_3 = 0.5$ and $R_3/R_1 = 2.8$. In practice, this choice of R_1 is limited somewhat by the requirement that the meter resistance be much higher than R_1; this makes R_1 a relatively small resistance.

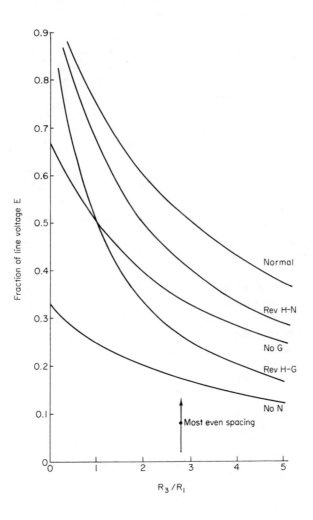

Fig. I-3 Variation of indications with R_3/R_1 (3-resistance technique). $R_2/R_3 = 0.5$.

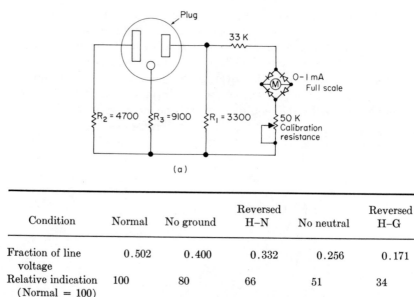

(a)

Condition	Normal	No ground	Reversed H–N	No neutral	Reversed H–G
Fraction of line voltage	0.502	0.400	0.332	0.256	0.171
Relative indication (Normal = 100)	100	80	66	51	34

(b)

Fig. I-4 Practical 3-resistance-technique circuit. (a) High-impedance metering using a rectifier bridge, a dc meter, and a calibration resistance has a negligible effect on R_1, R_2, R_3. (b) Indications obtained are well separated and allow for ±10% tolerance variations on components.

A practical implementation might be as shown in Fig. I-4a, which uses a rectifier bridge to convert the ac so that a 0–1-mA dc meter movement can be used. Also shown in Fig. I-4b are the meter indications for each condition. With this arrangement, component variations up to 10% are permissible before overlapping of fault regions on the meter can occur.

Appendix J

BIOMEDICAL EQUIPMENT TECHNICIAN

Education

1. The BMET should have an Associate of Arts Degree in Applied Science or equivalent.
2. He or she must understand the theory of operation of the following:

   (1) Multigun and storage oscilloscopes
   (2) Digital voltmeters and digital counters
   (3) Variable-frequency generators
   (4) D'Arsonval meters and LED meter displays
   (5) Squirrel-cage, synchro, and servo motors
   (6) Electronic regulated power supplies with remote programming
   (7) Differential amplifiers and white noise
   (8) Radio-frequency circuitry
   (9) Complex timer circuitry for synchronization.

3. He or she must have a good working knowledge of algebra, trigonometry, and plane geometry.

Duties

1. Assists physicians in setting up and operating specialized electronic equipment.
2. Carries out preventive maintenance program, as delineated by biomedical instrumentation engineer (BMIE) involving complex testing and calibration of sophisticated medical instrumentation.

3. Instructs doctors, nurses, and medical technicians in proper use and care of instrumentation, as outlined by BMIE.
4. Evaluates new equipment according to methods delineated by BMIE.
5. Constructs and tests complex prototype equipment from design schematics and sketches supplied by BMIE.
6. Makes repairs to and modifies equipment and instrumentation as required.
7. Trouble-shoots complex solid-state and vacuum-tube circuitry.
8. Must maintain a uniform PM record system and work status log.

Responsibilities

1. Is held responsible to BMIE for patient safety via safety tests (leakage, grounding, etc.) on equipment.
2. Takes risks in testing high-voltage electrosurgical devices, ultrasonic therapy machines, diathermy machines, and defibrillators.
3. Must work in OR, ICU, or CCU as may be required under emergency and/or adverse conditions.
4. Is held responsible to BMIE for reports on equipment condition and work status.

Appendix K

APPLICATION OF THÉVENIN'S
THEOREM TO A GROUND MONITOR

Consider the ground monitor shown in Fig. K-1. Consider first that only load Z_{L1} is connected to the circuit (i.e., load Z_{L2} is not connected to the circuit). Furthermore, switch S is connected to the junction of Z_1 and Z_2 for the purpose of this analysis. What is the current through Z_{L1}?

This part of the problem has already been partially discussed in Chapter 2, where it was pointed out that under those conditions the open circuit voltage across terminals a–a' would be given by $E\,Z_1/(Z_1 + Z_2)$, and the impedance looking into terminals a–a' would be given by Z_5 in series with Z_1 and Z_2 in parallel, or $[Z_1 \cdot Z_2/(Z_1 + Z_2)] + Z_5$. The equivalent circuit of this configuration is that shown in Fig. 2-23 and also in Fig. K-2.

If a fault load Z_{L1} arises, the current flowing through it will be given by

$$I_{ZL1} = \frac{E[Z_1/(Z_1 + Z_2)]}{[Z_1 Z_2/(Z_1 + Z_2)] + Z_5 + Z_{L1}}$$

If switch S is switched from terminal 1 to terminal 2, Z_3 and Z_4 are substituted, respectively, for Z_1 and Z_2.

Referring again to Fig. K-1, what is the current through Z_{L1} if a fault load Z_{L2} arises also?

The analysis of this latter situation is little more complicated. Again, we have to find (a) the open-circuit voltage V across terminals a–a' with Z_{L2} connected but Z_{L1} disconnected, and (b) short-circuit the voltage source E, and find the impedance looking into terminals a–a'.

The new equivalent circuit, as far as finding the voltage across terminals a–a' is concerned, is illustrated in Fig. K-3. To find voltage V, we proceed to first find voltage V_1, which is the ratio of the voltage developed across Z_1 compared to the voltage developed across the impedance that E

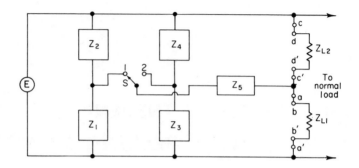

Fig. K-1 Ground monitor with fault loads.

is looking into multiplied by E, and is consequently E multiplied by the ratio of impedance Z_1 to the combined impedance presented by impedances Z_1, Z_{L2}, Z_5, and Z_2 connected as shown in Fig. K-3. Thus V_1 is now

$$V_1 = E\,\frac{Z_1(Z_2 + Z_5 + Z_{L2})}{Z_{L2}(Z_1 + Z_2) + Z_1(Z_5 + Z_2 Z_5 + Z_1 Z_2)}$$

Next we proceed to find the total current I_t through the combined impedances of Z_1, Z_{L2}, Z_5, and Z_2, connected as shown, which is given by

$$I_t = E\,\frac{Z_2 + Z_5 + Z_{L2}}{Z_{L2}(Z_1 + Z_2) + Z_1 Z_5 + Z_2 Z_5 + Z_1 Z_2}$$

This total current I_t divides respectively into a current I_{Z1} flowing through Z_1 and into a current $I_{ZL2,Z5}$, flowing through impedances Z_{L2} and Z_5 in series. The magnitudes of the currents in these two branches are inversely proportional to the impedances presented by the branches, and consequently

$$I_{ZL2,Z5} = E\,\frac{Z_2}{Z_{L2} + Z_5 + Z_2}\cdot\frac{Z_2 + Z_5 + Z_{L2}}{Z_{L2}(Z_1 + Z_2) + Z_1 Z_5 + Z_2 Z_5 + Z_1 Z_2}$$

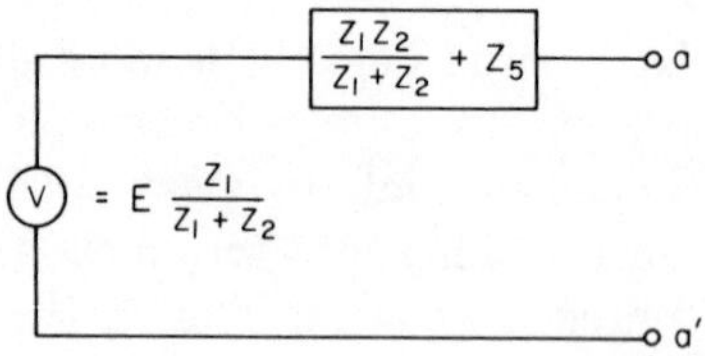

Fig. K-2 Equivalent circuit of Fig. 1 with terminals a–a′ and c–c′ open-circuited.

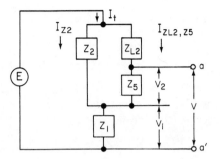

Fig. K-3 Equivalent circuit of Fig. K-1 for finding voltage V across terminals a–a', terminals c–c' being connected to load Z_{L2}.

The voltage V_2 across impedance Z_5 is given by $I_{Z_{L2},Z_5} \times Z_5$, i.e.,

$$V_2 = E \frac{Z_2 Z_5}{Z_{L2} + Z_5 + Z_i} \cdot \frac{Z_2 + Z_5 + Z_{L2}}{Z_{L2}(Z_1 + Z_2) + Z_1 Z_5 + Z_2 Z_5 + Z_1 Z_2}$$

and

$$V = V_1 + V_2$$

or

$$V = E \frac{Z_2 Z_5 + Z_1(Z_{L2} + Z_5 + Z_2)}{Z_{L2}(Z_1 + Z_2) + Z_1 Z_5 + Z_2 Z_5 + Z_1 Z_2}$$

The equivalent circuit for finding the impedance looking into terminals a–a' is shown in Fig. K-4. From the circuit configuration, it can be de-

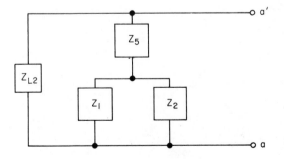

Fig. K-4 Equivalent circuit of Fig. K-1 with no fault loads looking into terminals a–a'.

termined that the impedance $Z_{a-a'}$ is given by

$$Z_{a-a'} = \frac{(Z_5Z_1 + Z_2Z_5 + Z_1Z_2)Z_{L2}}{(Z_1 + Z_2) \cdot (Z_{L2} + Z_5) + Z_1Z_2}$$

It is interesting to note that when Z_{L2} tends to infinity, which is equivalent to saying that Z_{L2} is mathematically taken out of the circuit, so to speak, $Z_{a-a'}$ reduces to the former expression

$$[(Z_1 \cdot Z_2)/(Z_1 + Z_2)] + Z_5$$

and likewise V reduces to the former expression $E Z_1/(Z_1 + Z_2)$. This can readily be verified by ignoring all terms that are small in comparison to Z_{L2}, and then equating the ratio $Z_{L2}/Z_{L2} = 1$.

The current through Z_{L1} when switch S is in position 1 and impedances Z_1 and Z_2 are in the circuit is then given by

$$I_{ZL1(Z_1,Z_2)} = \frac{V}{Z_{a-a'} + Z_{L1}}$$

which will, among other terms, contain the terms Z_1 and Z_2.

When switch S is in position 2, Z_3 and Z_4 are substituted for Z_1 and Z_2, respectively, to obtain $I_{ZL1(Z_3,Z_4)}$. The average fault current through $ZL1$ is then given by

$$I_{ZL1(av)} = \frac{I_{ZL1(Z_1,Z_2)} + I_{ZL1(Z_3,Z_4)}}{2}$$

Appendix L

NPN TRANSISTOR LOAD LINE

For typical output characteristics of an NPN transistor with both varying base currents and varying collector-to-emitter voltages, refer to Fig. 2-29 in Chapter 2.

Line A-B on Fig. 2-29 is called the load line of the transistor. Assume that a base current of 200 μA flows in the base of the transistor. Then the collector of the transistor, i.e., point c of Fig. 2-27, will assume a voltage of approximately 13 V, as seen from point Q of Fig. 2-29, and the current flowing in the load resistor R_L and the base resistor R_B of Fig. 2-27 will be 15 mA at this point. If the load current is decreased to 0 μA, the voltage of the collector will rise to approximately 21 V (point R of Fig. 2-29), and if the base current is raised to 400 μA, the voltage of the collector will drop to 6 V (point P of Fig. 2-29). A swing of 200 μA in either direction in the base current, i.e., from 200 down to zero and then up again to 400 μA will result in a corresponding voltage swing of the collector from 13 V at 15 mA (point Q) up to 21 V at 5 mA (point R) and down again to 6 V at 22 mA (point Q), or a total swing of (21 − 6) = 15 V.

Thus for an input current swing of ± 200 μA we have been able to obtain a voltage output swing of ± 7.5 V, or a total current swing of (22 − 5) = 17 mA, corresponding to a ±8.5 mA current swing in the output circuit, or a current gain of 8.5 mA/200 μA = 42.5 caused by the gain in the transistor which converted a small current swing in the base to a large current or voltage swing across the transistor load R_L. The foregoing analysis has covered dc gain characteristics of the transistor, since the direct currents occurring in the transistor in the NPN configuration have already been discussed. It should be noted that the load line previously mentioned corresponds to a total dc circuit resistance of 25 V/30 mA = 833 ohms, and the intersection of the load line with the voltage and current axes yields the 25 V and 30 mA points B and A, respectively. The resistance of 833 ohms is made up of both the load resistance R_L and the base resistance R_b in series.

INDEX

A 5
B 6
C 7
D 8
E 9
F 0
G 1
H 2
I 3
J 4